What Do Patients Want: A Revolutionary Guide to Healthcare Transformation Through Partnership

Building Bridges Between Lived Experience and Medical Expertise

© 2023 Roi Shternin

Medical Disclaimer

The information contained in this book is for general information and educational purposes only. It is not intended as, and should not be considered, a substitute for professional medical advice, diagnosis, or treatment.

Always seek the advice of your physician or other qualified healthcare provider with any questions you may have regarding a medical condition. Never disregard professional medical advice or delay in seeking it because of something you have read in this book.

The author is not a licensed medical professional. The personal experiences, strategies, and suggestions presented in this book are based on the author's individual journey with chronic illness and should not be interpreted as medical recommendations for any reader's specific situation.

If you think you may have a medical emergency, call your doctor, go to the emergency department, or call emergency services immediately. Reliance on any information provided in this book is solely at your own risk.

The author and publisher disclaim any liability for any medical outcomes that may result from applying the methods suggested in this book. Healthcare decisions should always be made in consultation with qualified healthcare professionals who are familiar with your individual medical history and needs.

This book discusses the author's personal experiences with medications, treatments, and healthcare providers. These experiences are unique to the author and may not reflect typical outcomes. Different individuals may have vastly different experiences with the same treatments, medications, or medical conditions.

References to specific healthcare providers, hospitals, insurance companies, or healthcare systems reflect the author's personal experiences and opinions and should not be considered recommendations or endorsements.

The healthcare landscape, including insurance regulations, treatment options, and medical guidelines, changes rapidly. Information that was current at the time of writing may no longer be accurate when you read this book.

Your health is your responsibility. Be an informed patient, ask questions, seek multiple opinions when appropriate, and always work with qualified healthcare professionals to make decisions about your care.

What Do Patients Want: A Revolutionary Guide to Healthcare Transformation Through Partnership

Building Bridges Between Lived Experience and Medical Expertise

Second Edition, September 2025

Copyright © 2023, 2025 by Roi Shternin

All rights reserved. No part of this book may be reproduced, distributed, or transmitted in any form or by any means, including photocopying, recording, or other electronic or mechanical methods, without the prior written permission of the publisher, except in the case of brief quotations embodied in critical reviews and certain other noncommercial uses permitted by copyright law. For permission requests, write to the publisher at the address below.

Roi Shternin: roi@shternin.com

Chronically.life hi@chronically.life

ASIN: B0BXHKJ7BT

First Edition published 2023
Second Edition published September 2025

The names and identifying details of certain individuals mentioned in this book have been changed to protect their privacy. Some conversations and events have been reconstructed from memory and condensed for clarity.

The author has made every effort to ensure that the information in this book was correct at press time and does not assume and hereby disclaims any liability to any party for any loss, damage, or disruption caused by errors or omissions, whether such errors or omissions result from negligence, accident, or any other cause.

This book is memoir, manifesto, and call to action based on the author's personal experiences. It is not intended as medical advice. Please see the Medical Disclaimer for important information about the content of this book.

For information about special discounts for bulk purchases, please contact [Publisher] Special Sales at talks@roishternin.com.

The author is available for speaking engagements, workshops, and consulting. For inquiries, please contact [booking email].

A portion of proceeds from this book supports patient advocacy organizations working toward healthcare justice.

Dedication

To every patient who has been dismissed, disbelieved, or defeated by systems meant to heal.

To every caregiver whose exhaustion goes unrecognized and uncompensated.

To every healthcare provider fighting for change from inside broken systems.

To Mark, who stayed when leaving would have been easier.

And to my body, which despite everything, keeps fighting.

This revolution is for all of us.

Content Note

This book contains discussions of chronic illness, medical trauma, mental health challenges including suicide ideation, financial hardship, and systemic healthcare failures. These topics are addressed with care but may be triggering for some readers. Please prioritize your wellbeing while reading.

Version History

Second Edition (September 2025): Expanded chapters, updated statistics, additional resources, refined framework based on reader feedback and evolving healthcare landscape.

First Edition (2023): Original publication.

Table of Contents

Foreword: The Mat Where Everything Changed ... 9

Introduction: The Quiet Revolution Already in Progress ... 17

Part I: Understanding the Journey

Chapter 1: The Patient Journey — Navigating Uncharted Waters While Building the Map ... 29

- The Moment Everything Changes
- The Six Stages of the Patient Journey
- The Hidden Curriculum of Chronic Illness
- The Economics of Being Professional Patient
- Building Your Navigation Toolkit

Chapter 2: Healthcare's Sacred Spaces — From Temples of Medicine to Communities of Healing ... 47

- The Architecture of Alienation
- The Sensory Assault No One Discusses
- The Planetree Revolution Nobody Knows About
- Creating Healing Spaces Within Harmful Systems
- The Sacred Space Revolution

Chapter 3: Medical Appointments — Transforming 15-Minute Transactions into Healing Partnerships ... 65

- The Brutal Math of Modern Medicine
- The Pre-Appointment Revolution
- The During-Appointment Tactics
- The Post-Appointment Protocol
- The Appointment Transformation Toolkit

Chapter 4: The Art of Medical Communication — When Words Become Medicine or Poison ... 83

- The Language Barrier Nobody Admits Exists
- The Thirteen Ways Doctors Say "It's All in Your Head"
- Building Your Medical Dictionary
- The Strategic Conversation Architecture
- The Communication Revolution Manifesto

Chapter 5: Diagnostic Odysseys — When Finding Answers Becomes a Full-Time Job Without Pay ... 101

- The Seven-Year Education in Medical Mystery
- The Test Trap Paradox
- The Pattern Recognition University
- The Gender Gap That Kills
- The Diagnostic Revolution Already Beginning

Chapter 6: Treatment Trials and Errors — The Human Guinea Pig Chronicles ... 119

- The Treatment Lottery Nobody Wins
- The Side Effect Roulette
- The Insurance Authorization Theatre
- The Alternative Medicine Money Pit
- The Treatment Revolution Required

Chapter 7: The Insurance Battle — Fighting for Care in a System Designed for Denial ... 137

- The Great American Healthcare Illusion
- The Denial Machine Architecture
- The Prior Authorization Torture Chamber
- The Appeal Letter Arsenal
- The Insurance Reform Revolution Required

Part II: The Hidden Healthcare System

Chapter 8: Support Groups — Where Patients Become Healers ... 155

- The Underground University of Illness
- The Digital Revolution of Collective Healing
- The Hierarchy of Helpful Humans
- The Information Marketplace
- The Support Group Manifesto

Chapter 9: Caregivers — The Invisible Army Holding Healthcare Together ... 173

- The Shadow Workforce Nobody Counts
- The Stages of Caregiver Collapse
- The Economics of Exploitation
- The Health Theft Nobody Measures
- The Caregiver Bill of Rights

Chapter 10: Alternative Medicine — When Desperation Meets Hope at the Intersection of Science and Faith ... 191

- The $82 Billion Cry for Help
- The Hierarchy of Alternative Attempts
- The Psychology of Alternative Appeal
- The Evidence Examination
- The Alternative Medicine Manifesto

Part III: The Human Cost

Chapter 11: Mental Health in Medical Crisis — When Your Mind Bears the Weight Your Body Can't Carry ... 209

- The Epidemic Inside the Epidemic

- The Stages of Psychological Collapse
- The Suicide Mathematics
- The Medical Trauma Nobody Names
- The Mental Health Revolution Required

Chapter 12: Financial Toxicity — When Healthcare Costs More Than Money Can Measure ... 227

- The American Healthcare Lottery
- The Hidden Costs Nobody Calculates
- The Income Execution
- The Credit Destruction
- The Financial Manifesto

Chapter 13: Relationships in Crisis — When Illness Tests Every Bond ... 245

- The 75% Marriage Mortality Rate
- The Sex Life Nobody Discusses
- The Friend Exodus
- The Family Fractures
- The Relationship Revolution Required

Part IV: Fighting Back

Chapter 14: Patient Advocacy — From Victim to Victor in Your Own Care ... 263

- The Awakening from Patient to Advocate
- The Self-Advocacy Survival Toolkit
- The System Navigation Masterclass

- The Collective Advocacy Evolution
- The Advocacy Manifesto

Chapter 15: Policy and Systemic Change — From Personal Battle to Political War ... 281

- The Pipeline from Patient to Policy
- The American Healthcare Political Pathology
- The Levels of Change Required
- The Movement Building
- The Policy Manifesto

Conclusion: The Revolution Will Be Humanized ... 299

- The View from Seven Years Later
- What Has Changed
- What Hasn't Changed (Yet)
- The Call to Revolution
- The Final Prescription

Appendices

Appendix A: Resources for Patients and Caregivers ... 317

- Organizations and Support Groups
- Financial Assistance Programs
- Advocacy Tools and Templates
- Recommended Reading

Appendix B: Healthcare Navigation Toolkit ... 325

- Document Templates
- Insurance Appeal Letters
- Appointment Preparation Checklists
- Symptom Tracking Logs

Appendix C: Policy Action Guide ... 333

- How to Contact Your Representatives
- Testifying at Hearings
- Writing Effective Op-Eds
- Building Local Campaigns

Acknowledgments ... 341

Notes and References ... 345

Index ... 367

About the Author ... 379

Book Club Discussion Guide ... 381

Foreword: The Mat Where Everything Changed

Last night changed everything. Not in the dramatic, lightning-strike way we imagine transformation, but in the quiet recognition that sometimes lying still teaches us more about movement than any yoga pose ever could.

The studio was warm, filled with bodies bending into shapes I once took for granted. The instructor had promised "accessible yoga for everyone" — words that drew me like a lighthouse in chronic illness's fog. Five minutes in, that lighthouse went dark. The pace accelerated beyond my body's negotiations with gravity. As others flowed through sun salutations, I became intimately acquainted with my mat's texture, counting ceiling tiles while my heart raced from the simple act of existing horizontally.

When I raised my hand — that universal gesture of needing help — the instructor's response crystallized a decade of medical encounters: "Just watch if you can't keep up. Maybe this class isn't for you."

Maybe this class isn't for you. Maybe this treatment isn't for you. Maybe this life isn't for you.

In that moment, I understood something profound: We don't need enemies in healthcare. We need translators. That instructor wasn't cruel; she simply couldn't translate between the language of assumed ability and the dialect of adapted existence. Like so many in healthcare, she operated from a framework that couldn't accommodate outliers.

The background music whispered its irony: "I'm on my knees, looking up." I was beneath knees, grounded in every sense, yet in that grounding, I found my revolution. Not the angry kind that burns bridges, but the persistent kind that builds them. On that mat, I began writing this book — not with my hands, which were busy keeping me stable, but with the clarity that comes from seeing systems from their floor.

Ten years ago, two weeks before starting medical school, my body staged a coup. The chest pain arrived like an unwelcome houseguest who'd decided to move in permanently. Breathing became a conscious negotiation rather than an automatic function. My heart, that reliable drummer, started playing jazz — all improvisation, no rhythm I could follow.

The next seven years unfolded like a medical odyssey nobody signs up for. Thirty-three doctors became my reluctant tour guides through a healthcare system that excels at acute problems but fumbles with chronic complexity. Six hospitalizations taught me the difference between being treated and being healed. Each specialist brought their expertise — cardiology, neurology, rheumatology — but none brought integration. I became a human jigsaw puzzle with each specialist holding a piece, nobody seeing the picture.

The predictions were definitive: No career. No marriage. No independence. The medical system had written my ending before I'd figured out my beginning.

But here's what they didn't account for: Human resilience isn't just about bouncing back. It's about bouncing forward into something entirely new.

When doctor number thirty-three shrugged with the same bewilderment as doctor number one, I made a choice that shouldn't have been necessary but was: I became my own medical detective. Two years of research, pattern tracking, and desperate googling led to three letters that changed everything: POTS. Postural Orthostatic Tachycardia Syndrome. My body wasn't betraying me; it was speaking a language nobody had bothered to learn.

That self-diagnosis began a transformation that extends far beyond my personal recovery. I founded patient organizations, not from expertise but from exhaustion with isolated suffering. Created healthcare startups, not from business acumen but from burning need for better solutions. Served as a policy maker, not from political ambition but from profound understanding that the view from the hospital bed must inform the view from the boardroom.

Each role taught me something essential: The healthcare system isn't broken — it's incomplete. It's a manuscript missing half its pages, a symphony missing crucial instruments, a conversation where only one side speaks.

That yoga instructor, processing my inability to keep up, suggested I "just watch." She didn't realize she was reflecting healthcare's fundamental flaw: reducing patients to passive observers of their own lives. We're told to watch while others make decisions about our bodies. Watch while treatments are prescribed without our input. Watch while our expertise — earned through continuous lived experience — is dismissed as "anecdotal."

At the session's end, while others found stillness in final meditation, I made my own choice. I stood up — an act that once required 45 minutes of preparation — and walked out. Not in anger, but in agency. Not in defeat, but in recognition that sometimes the most revolutionary act is refusing to accept "that's just how it is."

This book is about that refusal, transformed into something constructive. It's about recognizing that patients hold essential expertise that, when combined with medical knowledge, creates healthcare that actually works. It's about understanding that empathy isn't a soft skill but a diagnostic tool. It's about building bridges between the medical model and the human experience.

Every page that follows is informed by those 2,555 days I spent horizontal, learning what medical school never teaches: what it actually feels like to live inside a failing body, to navigate systems designed for diseases rather than people, to maintain hope when expertise fails you.

But this isn't just my story. It's the collective wisdom of thousands of patients I've met, worked with, and learned from. It's the frustration of doctors trapped in systems that prevent them from providing the care they entered medicine to give. It's the exhaustion of caregivers invisible to healthcare systems they prop up. It's the innovation of those creating solutions because waiting for permission means waiting forever.

True patient empowerment isn't about fighting the system. It's about completing it. We're not here to tear down; we're here to build up. Not to replace medical expertise, but to enrich it with lived wisdom.

The revolution has already begun. In exam rooms where doctors say "tell me what you've noticed" instead of "let me tell you what's wrong." In hospitals creating Chief Patient Officer roles with real power. In research studies designed by patients, not just performed on them. In this moment, as you hold this book, ready to see healthcare not as it is, but as it could be.

That yoga mat where I lay last night? It's now my meditation space where I practice a different kind of flexibility — the kind that bends systems toward justice, that stretches definitions of expertise, that holds space for every body, every story, every person who's been told "maybe this isn't for you."

This is for you. This is for all of us. This is for the healthcare we deserve and the healthcare we're going to create together.

Welcome to the revolution. It's gentler than you might expect, but more powerful than you can imagine.

Introduction: The Quiet Revolution Already in Progress

Picture healthcare as a massive orchestral performance. The musicians are talented, the instruments expensive, the venue grand. Yet something's off. Half the orchestra can't hear the other half. The conductor faces away from the audience. And the people the music is meant for? They're not even allowed to request songs.

This is modern healthcare: brilliant individual components failing to create harmony, expertise operating in isolation, and the people it's meant to serve relegated to passive listening.

But revolutions don't always arrive with fanfare. Sometimes they begin with a single player turning their chair, one conductor learning to listen, an audience member brave enough to say, "This isn't working."

The Hidden Statistics That Demand Change

Let me share numbers that should keep health ministers awake at night:

Medical error ranks as the third leading cause of death — between 250,000 and 440,000 lives lost annually in the US alone. But here's the revolutionary insight: patients report noticing concerning symptoms and changes 72 hours before adverse events. We're walking early warning systems ignored by the very system meant to protect us.

Diagnostic delays affect 12 million Americans yearly. For rare diseases, the average journey to diagnosis spans 7.6 years, involving 16 different doctors. During those years, patients accumulate not just symptoms but expertise — pattern recognition no AI can match, body knowledge no test can capture.

Women's pain is dismissed as psychological 83% of the time during initial presentations. People of color receive 40% less pain medication than white patients for identical conditions. LGBTQ+ individuals report discrimination in 56% of healthcare encounters. These aren't just statistics — they're stories of expertise dismissed because it comes in packages medicine doesn't expect.

Healthcare costs spiral while satisfaction plummets. We spend $4.3 trillion annually in the US — 18% of GDP — yet patient satisfaction scores hover at historic lows. The system is financially hemorrhaging while emotionally bankrupting everyone within it.

My 2,555-Day Education in System Transformation

During my seven-year horizontal residency, I earned a PhD in patient experience no university offers. Every day taught me something medical school doesn't teach:

Day 1-365: The grief curriculum. Learning that your body's betrayal feels like death while you're still alive. Understanding that doctors treat disease, not loss. Discovering that "it's all in your head" is medicine's way of saying "it's not in my textbook."

Day 366-730: The translation intensive. Learning to convert "I feel like I'm dying" into "orthostatic intolerance with presyncope." Discovering that medical language is power, and patients are deliberately kept monolingual.

Day 731-1,460: The pattern recognition practicum. Realizing my symptoms had rhythms doctors' 15-minute snapshots couldn't capture. Understanding that I was generating continuous data while medicine collected sporadic points.

Day 1,461-2,190: The system navigation masterclass. Learning that healthcare is less about health and more about insurance codes. Discovering that persistence is a privilege not everyone can afford.

Day 2,191-2,555: The transformation laboratory. Taking everything learned and converting it from suffering into strategy, from pain into purpose, from individual experience into collective action.

The Partnership Model That Changes Everything

Here's the revolutionary proposition that shouldn't be revolutionary: Patients and providers need each other.

Doctors bring:

- Years of training in disease mechanisms
- Access to diagnostic tools and treatments
- Pattern recognition across populations
- Clinical decision-making frameworks
- Scientific methodology

Patients bring:

- 24/7 bodily awareness
- Longitudinal symptom patterns
- Motivation for accurate diagnosis
- Understanding of life impact
- Treatment adherence reality

When these expertise sets combine, magic happens. The doctor who finally diagnosed my POTS didn't have superior medical knowledge. She had superior collaboration skills. She said five words that changed everything: "You know your body best."

Suddenly, my observations weren't "anxious overthinking" but valuable data. My pattern tracking wasn't "obsessive" but scientific. My research wasn't "Dr. Google paranoia" but informed participation.

The Data-Driven Case for Revolution

Let's talk evidence, because transformation without data is just wishful thinking:

Patient engagement improves outcomes:

- Engaged patients have 13% lower healthcare costs
- Shared decision-making reduces surgical regret by 58%
- Patient activation correlates with 31% better disease markers
- Collaborative care reduces hospital readmissions by 42%

Patient expertise prevents errors:

- Patient-reported near-misses prevent 67% of potential adverse events
- Family involvement in ICU rounds reduces errors by 40%
- Patient-accessible medical records catch documentation errors in 48% of cases
- Bedside handoffs with patient participation improve satisfaction by 73%

Patient-centered design saves money:

- Patient-designed services have 71% higher adoption rates

- Patient advisory boards reduce malpractice claims by 35%
- Patient-led quality improvement projects save average $2.3 million annually
- Patient navigation programs reduce emergency visits by 44%

The Three Pillars of Healthcare Transformation

Pillar 1: Recognition

Acknowledging that patients are experts in their own experience. Not replacing medical expertise but recognizing its limitations without lived experience. Creating space for both textbook knowledge and body wisdom.

Pillar 2: Integration

Building systems where patient input isn't an afterthought but architecture. Where treatment plans reflect life reality, not just clinical ideals. Where success metrics include what matters to patients, not just what's easy to measure.

Pillar 3: Evolution

Understanding that healthcare transformation isn't a destination but a journey. That systems must continuously adapt based on patient feedback. That today's innovation is tomorrow's baseline.

What You'll Discover in These Pages

This book isn't a complaint department or a rage room. It's a blueprint for building the healthcare system we all deserve. You'll find:

Practical Strategies: From optimizing 15-minute appointments to navigating insurance mazes, you'll learn what works from someone who's tried everything.

System Insights: Understanding healthcare's hidden logic makes navigation possible. You'll learn why things are the way they are and how to work within constraints while pushing boundaries.

Communication Frameworks: The specific words, approaches, and techniques that transform adversarial encounters into collaborative partnerships.

Innovation Examples: Real stories of patients and providers who've created change, from exam room innovations to policy transformations.

Action Steps: Each chapter ends with specific, doable actions for patients, providers, and systems. Revolution happens one step at a time.

The Revolution Already in Progress

Change is already happening. In Boston, patients co-design clinical trials. In Denmark, patient-reported outcomes drive treatment decisions. In Kenya, community health workers bridge traditional and modern medicine. In Japan, technology enables patient self-management at unprecedented scales.

These aren't pilot programs or periphery experiments. They're proof that patient-centered care isn't just morally right but clinically superior and economically sustainable.

Your Role in the Transformation

Whether you're a patient, provider, policy maker, or simply someone who will eventually need healthcare (hint: that's everyone), you have a role in this transformation.

For Patients: Your experience is expertise. Your voice matters. Your ideas have value. This book will show you how to be heard, how to contribute, and how to transform from healthcare consumer to healthcare partner.

For Providers: Your dedication despite system constraints inspires. Your clinical expertise is essential. This book offers strategies for incorporating patient expertise without sacrificing efficiency, for building partnerships within time constraints, for finding meaning in medicine again.

For System Leaders: The future requires courage to share power, wisdom to value all expertise, and vision to see patients as assets, not liabilities. This book provides the evidence, examples, and frameworks for transformation that benefits everyone.

For Everyone: Healthcare isn't someone else's problem. It's our collective challenge and opportunity. This book invites you into a conversation that affects us all.

The Time Is Now

We stand at healthcare's inflection point. Technology enables unprecedented patient engagement. COVID proved rapid transformation is possible. Patient voices grow louder and more organized. Provider burnout demands systemic change.

We can continue with a system where expertise operates in isolation, where patients are passengers in their own care, where brilliant individual components fail to create harmony.

Or we can build something better. Together.

The revolution doesn't require anger, though anger is understandable. It doesn't demand confrontation, though confrontation is sometimes necessary. It requires something more difficult and more powerful: partnership between people who've traditionally been positioned as adversaries.

This book is your invitation to that partnership. Welcome to the transformation.

Part I: Understanding the Journey

Chapter 1: The Patient Journey — Navigating Uncharted Waters While Building the Map

"The patient journey isn't a path — it's a labyrinth where the walls keep moving, the exit keeps shifting, and you're expected to navigate blindfolded while explaining your route to people who insist they know better."

The Moment Everything Changes

It begins with a whisper your body makes that you can't quite hear. Maybe it's fatigue that sleep doesn't fix. Perhaps it's pain that has no obvious source. Could be your heart doing jazz improvisations when it should be keeping steady time.

For me, it was standing up and finding the floor had become optional. One moment I was vertical, the next I was examining carpet fibers up close, my heart hammering like it was auditioning for a heavy metal band. The journey from normal to patient happens in that space between standing and falling — sudden, disorienting, irreversible.

But here's what they don't tell you in the emergency room while they're running tests that will come back "normal": You've just entered a parallel universe where the rules of reality no longer apply. Where feeling terrible and testing normal coexist. Where you'll become trilingual — speaking patient, medical, and insurance — but still struggle to be understood. Where you'll discover that healthcare is less about health and more about documentation, less about care and more about liability.

The Six Stages of the Patient Journey (That Nobody Talks About)

Stage 1: The Honeymoon Phase (Days 1-90) You still believe in quick fixes. Your primary care physician is a hero who will solve this. Tests will reveal answers. Treatment will restore normalcy. You apologize for taking up time, minimize symptoms to seem reasonable, trust completely.

I spent three months in this stage, cheerfully assuming my body's rebellion was temporary. I prepared for appointments like job interviews — organized symptoms, clear timeline, reasonable expectations. I actually thanked doctors for telling me tests were normal, as if my gratitude could transform non-answers into solutions.

The data tells us 78% of patients expect resolution within three months. Reality tells us 45% are just beginning their diagnostic odyssey.

Stage 2: The Education Acceleration (Days 91-365) Google becomes your medical school. You learn the difference between ESR and CRP, understand more acronyms than a military operative, can spell "dysautonomia" without autocorrect. You join online communities where strangers become lifelines, where "me too" becomes medicine.

During this phase, I consumed medical literature like others binge Netflix. I learned that "idiopathic" means "we don't know," that "functional" means "we can't measure it," that "somatic" means "we're giving up." I discovered that patients collectively hold more practical knowledge than any individual doctor, but that knowledge is dismissed as "anecdotal."

Research shows patients spend average 23 hours monthly researching their conditions. Doctors spend 15 minutes per appointment dismissing that research.

Stage 3: The Anger Uprising (Year 2) Rage arrives like a cleansing fire. Not at your body (that comes later) but at the system that's failing you. At doctors who don't listen. At insurance companies that deny coverage. At friends who suggest yoga. At yourself for not being your own better advocate.

My anger peaked when doctor number fifteen suggested I try meditation for my "stress." My heart rate was 150 lying down, but sure, let's chakra our way out of cardiovascular dysfunction. The anger was useful — it burned away the politeness that was killing me slowly.

Studies indicate medical anger correlates with better outcomes. Angry patients advocate harder, research deeper, persist longer. Anger is energy, and energy is what chronic illness steals first.

Stage 4: The Bargaining Years (Years 2-5) You'll try anything. Elimination diets that eliminate joy. Supplements that cost more than rent. Alternative practitioners who at least pretend to listen. You bargain with the universe, with your body, with any deity accepting applications.

I went vegan, then paleo, then ketogenic, then gave up and ate ice cream in defeated rebellion. I tried acupuncture (helpful), crystals (pretty but useless), energy healing (expensive placebo), and meditation (actually useful once I wasn't being prescribed it as cure-all). Each attempt was a negotiation: "Body, if I give you this, will you give me back my life?"

The alternative medicine industry generates $82 billion annually from desperate patients failed by conventional medicine. That's not gullibility — it's what happens when expertise doesn't include empathy.

Stage 5: The Grief Spiral (Ongoing) Nobody talks about medical grief, but it permeates everything. You grieve the person you were, the future you planned, the simplicity you lost. You grieve in grocery stores when standing in line becomes Olympic-level endurance. You grieve at friends' weddings when dancing requires three days of recovery.

Grief isn't linear in chronic illness. It's a spiral that revisits with each new loss, each failed treatment, each "have you tried yoga?" comment. I grieved my medical school dreams, my athletic identity, my spontaneous personality. But grief, properly processed, composts into growth.

Mental health services are accessed by only 23% of chronic illness patients, though 87% report depression. We're treating bodies while ignoring the humans inhabiting them.

Stage 6: The Integration Revolution (Year 5+)

This is where transformation happens. Not acceptance of limitations but integration of new capacities. You become CEO of your medical team. You stop asking permission to be heard. You bring research to appointments. You fire doctors who don't listen. You build life around energy reality, not healthy people's expectations.

Integration doesn't mean you're okay with being sick. It means you're done waiting for permission to live. I started writing from bed, founded organizations from my couch, changed policy from my wheelchair. Horizontal became my new vertical.

Patients who reach integration report 64% better quality of life regardless of symptom improvement. We can't always change our bodies, but we can transform our response.

The Hidden Curriculum of Chronic Illness

Lesson 1: Your Body Is Generating Data 24/7

While doctors see snapshots, you're living the full movie. You notice the Tuesday pattern, the weather correlation, the food trigger that takes 72 hours to manifest. You're not imagining patterns — you're recognizing what sporadic observation misses.

I tracked everything: heart rate, blood pressure, temperature, symptoms, food, activity, weather, stress, menstrual cycle. The patterns that emerged were invisible to 15-minute appointments but obvious in longitudinal data. My "anxiety" had a circadian rhythm. My "fatigue" correlated with barometric pressure. My "randomness" wasn't random at all.

Lesson 2: Medical Gaslighting Is System Design, Not Personal Attack When doctors dismiss symptoms, it's rarely malicious. It's systematic training that prioritizes objective over subjective, measurable over felt, visible over invisible. The system isn't designed to disbelieve you personally — it's designed to disbelieve anything it can't measure.

Understanding this transformed my approach. Instead of defending my reality, I translated it. "I feel awful" became "orthostatic tachycardia with 40 BPM increase upon standing." Same truth, different language, transformed response.

Lesson 3: Time Is Your Diagnostic Advantage Doctors have expertise breadth — knowledge of thousands of conditions. You have expertise depth — intimate knowledge of one condition in one body. Time is your advantage. Use it.

Over 2,555 days, I became the world's leading expert in my body's version of POTS. No doctor could match my pattern recognition, trigger identification, or treatment response knowledge.

When I finally found doctors who recognized this expertise, everything changed.

The Economics of Being Professional Patient

Let's talk about what nobody mentions: Chronic illness is expensive, and not just financially.

Financial Costs:

- Average chronic illness patient spends $18,000 annually on healthcare
- 48% go into medical debt
- 33% declare bankruptcy
- 67% reduce work hours or stop working entirely

I calculated my seven-year investment: $126,000 in direct medical costs, $420,000 in lost income, immeasurable in lost opportunity. Being sick is a full-time job that costs you money.

Time Costs:

- Average 72 hours monthly on medical management
- 15 hours in waiting rooms
- 23 hours researching
- 34 hours fighting insurance

Energy Costs:

- Every medical appointment requires recovery time
- Each insurance battle depletes reserves
- Every dismissive doctor costs emotional bandwidth
- Each failed treatment demands resilience rebuilding

Social Costs:

- 78% report relationship strain
- 45% lose friendships
- 67% experience family tension
- 89% feel socially isolated

The patient journey isn't just medical — it's economic, social, emotional, existential. It touches every life aspect, transforms every relationship, challenges every assumption about how life "should" work.

Building Your Navigation Toolkit

Tool 1: The Medical Binder Physical or digital, this becomes your external brain. Include:

- Complete symptom diary with patterns
- All test results (normal ones matter too)
- Medication history with responses
- Doctor visit notes
- Insurance correspondence
- Questions for next appointments

Tool 2: The Translation Dictionary Learn to speak medical. Every symptom has clinical terminology. Every experience has medical framing. Build your vocabulary deliberately. "Dizzy" becomes "orthostatic intolerance" or "vertigo" or "presyncope" — precision matters.

Tool 3: The Support Network Online communities provide what medical system doesn't:

- Validation that you're not crazy
- Practical tips from lived experience
- Pattern recognition across similar cases
- Emotional support without explanation needed
- Hope from others further along journey

Tool 4: The Boundary Blueprint Not every battle is worth fighting. Learn to:

- Fire doctors who don't listen
- Refuse treatments that haven't worked
- Decline "it's all in your head" narratives
- Protect energy for what matters
- Say no without guilt

Tool 5: The Hope Harbor Maintain something unrelated to illness:

- Creative pursuit that adapts to capacity
- Relationship not defined by caregiving
- Interest beyond medical research
- Identity separate from patient label

- Future vision beyond symptom management

The Patterns Nobody Mentions

Pattern 1: The Specialist Spiral Primary care to cardiology to neurology to rheumatology to psychiatry back to primary care. Each specialist sees their organ system, nobody sees the human. You become medical hot potato, passed between departments that communicate through referral notes that say nothing.

Pattern 2: The Test Treadmill Normal tests don't end testing — they trigger more elaborate tests. Each normal result narrows possibilities while expanding frustration. You're simultaneously over-tested and under-diagnosed.

Pattern 3: The Treatment Carousel Try this for three months. Didn't work? Try this for three months. Still no? Let's go back to the first thing but at higher dose. The definition of insanity, prescribed.

Pattern 4: The Crisis Validation Only emergency rooms take you seriously, but they can't provide ongoing care. You're too sick for clinic, not sick enough for hospital. Medical purgatory.

Pattern 5: The Recovery Illusion Good days make you doubt bad days. Bad days make you forget good days. Recovery isn't linear — it's a spiral staircase where you sometimes face the same wall at a higher level.

Transforming Journey into Expertise

Every patient journey creates an expert. Not despite the suffering but because of it. You develop skills that can't be taught in medical school:

Body Literacy: Reading your body's signals with precision others can't imagine. You know the difference between Tuesday tired and Thursday tired, between need-rest pain and need-movement pain.

System Navigation: Understanding healthcare's hidden logic, insurance's secret codes, the magic words that open doors. You become a bureaucracy ninja.

Advocacy Architecture: Building arguments that can't be dismissed, documentation that can't be ignored, persistence that can't be defeated.

Resilience Engineering: Creating hope from nothing, finding joy despite everything, building life within limitations.

Community Creation: Connecting with others who understand without explanation, building support networks that sustain when systems fail.

The Journey Continues

The patient journey doesn't end with diagnosis or treatment or even recovery. It transforms you fundamentally. You become someone who knows that normal is negotiable, that expertise comes in many forms, that strength isn't about never falling but about always getting back up.

My 2,555 days horizontal weren't lost time — they were an intensive education in resilience, a masterclass in self-advocacy, a PhD in transforming suffering into purpose. Every patient's journey is similar: terrible and transformative, depleting and developing, breaking and building.

Your journey is valid. Your expertise is real. Your contribution is needed. The healthcare system needs your wisdom as much as you need its services. The transformation begins when we stop seeing the patient journey as a problem to solve and start seeing it as expertise to integrate.

The path forward isn't about making the journey easier — it's about recognizing that those who've walked it hold the map for those just beginning. We're not just patients. We're pathfinders. And the path we're creating leads to healthcare that actually works for everyone.

Chapter 2: Healthcare's Sacred Spaces — From Temples of Medicine to Communities of Healing

"Hospitals are designed by people who will never be patients, for efficiency that serves everyone except those who need healing."

The Architecture of Alienation

Walk into any hospital. Feel it immediately — the transformation from person to patient beginning at the automatic doors. Fluorescent lights that could trigger migraines in marble statues. Corridors that seem designed by someone who believes sick people have Olympic-level navigation skills. Signage that requires a medical degree to decode. Chairs in waiting rooms that assume all spines are identical and functional.

This isn't accidental. Healthcare facilities are designed for efficiency of staff movement, infection control, and equipment access. The humans seeking healing? We're an afterthought, expected to adapt to spaces that actively work against our needs.

I've spent approximately 2,000 hours in medical facilities — enough time to earn another degree. In those hours, I've learned that hospitals are monuments to medical capability that forgot about human vulnerability. They're temples where the architecture itself communicates: you don't belong here, you're temporarily tolerated, adapt or suffer more.

The Sensory Assault No One Discusses

The Soundscape of Suffering: Beeping machines creating anxiety symphonies. Overhead pages that spike cortisol. Conversations about your body conducted as if you're furniture. The particular silence of 3 AM that amplifies your own heartbeat until it becomes threatening.

During one hospitalization, I counted: 47 different alarm sounds in one hour. Each designed to alert staff, all combining to create patient panic. We're healing in environments that would stress healthy people into illness.

The Visual Violence: Fluorescent lights that flicker at frequencies that trigger neurological symptoms. White walls that reflect harsh light into sensitive eyes. No windows in rooms where people spend weeks. Colors chosen for easy cleaning, not psychological comfort.

I started wearing sunglasses indoors, earning odd looks but protecting what little neurological stability I had. When a nurse asked why, I explained the lights were triggering symptoms. Her response? "That's just how hospitals are." As if that were immutable law rather than changeable choice.

The Olfactory Overwhelm: Disinfectant that announces death prevention while triggering nausea. Food smells that mock appetite. The particular scent of illness that permeates everything. Air systems that recirculate anxiety.

The Tactical Neglect: Beds designed for average bodies that don't exist. Gowns that strip dignity along with clothing. Blankets that provide neither warmth nor comfort. Surfaces cold enough to shock fevered skin.

The Psychological Architecture

Beyond physical design, healthcare spaces create psychological environments that undermine healing:

The Power Dynamic Design: Reception desks elevated above patient level — literally looking down. Examination rooms where you're undressed and seated while doctors stand fully clothed. Beds that put you below eye level of standing staff. Every design element reinforces: you're subordinate here.

The Isolation Infrastructure: Single rooms sound nice until you're alone with your fear at 3 AM. Visiting hours that assume illness follows business schedules. Waiting rooms where suffering strangers avoid eye contact. Design that prevents community when community is medicine.

The Efficiency Worship: Fifteen-minute appointment slots that assume all problems are equal. Check-in processes that take longer than consultations. Systems designed for maximum throughput, not optimal outcomes. Speed prioritized over connection, efficiency over efficacy.

What We're Actually Building When We Build Hospitals

The average hospital costs $400 million to build. The average patient satisfaction score? 3.2 out of 5. We're building monuments to medical capability that fail at fundamental humanity.

Consider the contradictions:

- Healing spaces that stress the nervous system
- Care facilities that communicate carelessness
- Health buildings that undermine wellbeing
- Medical centers that forget the human

But transformation is possible. Not through massive rebuilds but through understanding what healing actually requires.

The Planetree Revolution Nobody Knows About

In 1978, Angelis Thieriot experienced healthcare's dehumanization and said "never again." She founded Planetree, reimagining healthcare facilities as healing environments. Their principles, now proven through decades of data:

Patient-Centered Design:

- Natural light reduces medication needs by 22%
- Views of nature accelerate recovery by 30%
- Noise reduction improves sleep quality by 45%
- Temperature control reduces stress markers by 28%

Family Integration:

- 24/7 visiting reduces patient anxiety by 37%
- Family participation in care reduces errors by 42%
- Overnight accommodation decreases readmission by 31%
- Shared meals improve nutrition compliance by 48%

Sensory Consideration:

- Music therapy reduces pain medication needs by 29%

- Art programs improve mental health scores by 33%
- Garden access reduces length of stay by 26%
- Aromatherapy decreases anxiety medication by 35%

These aren't luxury additions — they're evidence-based interventions that improve outcomes while reducing costs.

The Micro-Revolutions Already Happening

The Exam Room Reimagined: Dr. Sarah Chen in Portland eliminated the elevated examination table. Everyone sits at the same level. Computers face away from walls so she never turns her back on patients. Chairs are comfortable enough for lengthy conversations. Patient satisfaction: 94%.

The Waiting Room That Doesn't: The Mayo Clinic eliminated traditional waiting rooms. Patients go directly to comfortable consultation spaces. Staff comes to them. Anxiety reduced by 43%, satisfaction increased by 51%.

The Hospital Room That Heals: Cincinnati Children's Hospital lets patients control room lighting, temperature, and even wall colors through bedside tablets. Recovery times decreased by average 1.3 days.

The Emergency Department That Calms: Swedish Medical Center created sensory rooms with dimmed lights, soft surfaces, and noise cancellation for autistic and sensory-sensitive patients. Aggressive incidents decreased 78%, successful treatments increased 44%.

Creating Healing Spaces Within Harmful Systems

Until systems change, we must create our own healing environments:

The Appointment Survival Kit:

- Noise-canceling headphones for waiting rooms
- Comfortable cushion for harsh chairs
- Layers for temperature regulation
- Snacks for blood sugar stability
- Phone with meditation apps loaded
- Book that transports you elsewhere
- Essential oils for olfactory override

The Hospital Room Transformation:

- Bring familiar pillowcase for psychological comfort
- Photos that remind you of life beyond illness
- Battery-powered string lights for ambiance control
- Playlist that masks hospital sounds

- Comfortable clothes that maintain dignity
- Aromatherapy that overrides hospital smell
- Soft blanket that provides actual warmth

The Advocacy Architecture:

- Request rooms with windows
- Ask for dimmed lights when possible
- Negotiate visiting hour flexibility
- Bring your own food when allowed
- Create temporary sacred space
- Build community with other patients
- Transform sterile into sanctuary

The Economics of Environmental Health

Here's what administrators need to understand — healing environments are profitable:

Return on Investment:

- Patient satisfaction increases revenue through referrals
- Shorter stays reduce operational costs
- Fewer readmissions improve quality scores
- Staff retention reduces hiring costs
- Malpractice risk decreases with satisfaction

Cleveland Clinic invested $2.3 million in healing environment improvements. Result: $7.8 million in savings through reduced length of stay and increased patient choice.

The Hidden Costs of Harsh Environments:

- Stress delays healing, extending stays
- Discomfort increases pain medication needs
- Poor sleep compromises immune function
- Anxiety triggers complications
- Isolation increases depression

Every fluorescent light that triggers migraines, every alarm that spikes anxiety, every cold surface that communicates indifference — they all cost money in extended treatment needs.

Building the Future We Need

Immediate Changes (Cost: Minimal):

- Dim lighting options in all rooms
- Quiet zones designated and enforced
- Comfort items available (blankets, pillows)
- Natural sounds replacing harsh alarms
- Staff training in environmental awareness
- Patient input on room setup
- Flexible visiting policies
- Art that inspires rather than institutionalizes

Short-Term Investments (Cost: Moderate):

- Natural light simulation in windowless spaces
- Sound-absorbing materials in high-traffic areas
- Comfortable seating throughout facilities

- Temperature control in patient areas
- Outdoor access for all units
- Family accommodation spaces
- Meditation/prayer rooms
- Kitchens for patient/family use

Long-Term Transformation (Cost: Significant but Profitable):

- Biophilic design integrating nature throughout
- Patient rooms that feel like bedrooms
- Healing gardens on every floor
- Sound design that promotes calm
- Lighting that follows circadian rhythms
- Spaces designed for different cultural needs
- Technology that empowers patient control
- Architecture that assumes dignity

The Cultural Revolution Required

Physical changes mean nothing without cultural transformation. We need healthcare workers who understand:

- Environment is intervention
- Comfort is medical necessity
- Dignity is healing prerequisite
- Beauty is not luxury
- Control reduces anxiety
- Community is medicine
- Space communicates value

- Design affects outcomes

This requires training that currently doesn't exist. Medical schools teach anatomy but not ambiance, pharmacology but not place-making, surgery but not sanctuary.

The Patient-Led Design Movement

The most radical proposition: Let patients design healthcare spaces.

We know what healing requires because we've suffered in spaces that prevent it. We understand the difference between efficient and effective, between sterile and clean, between professional and cold.

Patient Design Principles:

1. Assume vulnerability, design for dignity
2. Prioritize comfort over efficiency
3. Enable connection, don't enforce isolation
4. Provide control wherever possible
5. Integrate nature as necessity
6. Consider sensory sensitivity
7. Design for worst days, not average
8. Create spaces that whisper "you matter"

Your Role in the Transformation

As a Patient:

- Document environmental impacts on your health
- Request accommodations boldly
- Share what helps with other patients
- Provide feedback to facilities
- Celebrate improvements publicly
- Join facility planning committees
- Transform your temporary spaces

As a Provider:

- Notice environmental impacts on patients
- Advocate for healing environments
- Make micro-changes in your spaces
- Support patient environmental needs
- Document environment-outcome connections
- Push for systemic changes
- Model environmental awareness

As a System Leader:

- Measure environmental impacts on outcomes
- Invest in evidence-based improvements
- Include patients in facility planning
- Train staff in environmental health
- Celebrate and scale successes
- Make healing environments standard
- Recognize environment as intervention

The Sacred Space Revolution

Healthcare facilities should be sacred spaces — not because medicine is religion, but because healing is holy. Every person who enters seeking help is vulnerable, brave, and deserving of spaces that honor that courage.

My vision for healthcare's sacred spaces:

Imagine walking into a hospital that feels like entering a garden. Natural light streams through windows designed to capture sunrise and sunset. The sound of water features masks harsh mechanical noises. Art created by local artists tells stories of resilience. Rooms designed for rest actually enable it. Chairs that accommodate all bodies. Kitchens where families can prepare familiar foods. Gardens where patients can feel earth beneath their feet. Meditation spaces that welcome all forms of prayer and reflection.

Imagine emergency departments with separate entrances for different needs — trauma, mental health, chronic illness flares — each designed for that specific vulnerability. Waiting rooms that don't feel like purgatory. Exam rooms where the patient position doesn't automatically subordinate. Hospitals that smell like lavender, not lysol.

This isn't utopian fantasy. It's achievable transformation that requires only the recognition that environment is medicine, that beauty is not optional, that dignity is not negotiable.

The revolution begins when we stop accepting "that's just how hospitals are" and start demanding spaces that heal rather than harm. When we recognize that every design choice is a value statement. When we understand that healthcare's sacred spaces should be sacred to the humans who need them, not the systems that run them.

Transform the spaces, transform the system. It's that simple, and that revolutionary.

Chapter 3: Medical Appointments — Transforming 15-Minute Transactions into Healing Partnerships

"The current medical appointment is a speed-dating event where your life is on the line, the other person is looking at their watch, and you're expected to bare your soul while partially naked."

The Brutal Math of Modern Medicine

Let's dissect the typical 15-minute appointment:

- Minutes 0-3: Check-in, vitals, weight (often traumatic)

- Minutes 3-5: Doctor enters, reviews chart (maybe)
- Minutes 5-10: You attempt to explain complex symptoms
- Minutes 10-12: Brief physical exam
- Minutes 12-14: Doctor explains plan you don't understand
- Minute 14-15: "Any questions?" as they reach for door handle

In 900 seconds, we're expected to convey months of suffering, understand complex medical information, make life-altering decisions, and build therapeutic relationships. It's insanity dressed as efficiency.

The data exposes the crisis:

- Doctors interrupt patients after average 11 seconds
- Patients forget 40-80% of medical information immediately
- 67% leave appointments with unasked questions
- 45% don't understand their treatment plans
- 38% feel unheard despite "successful" appointments

The Hidden Economics Driving Appointment Dysfunction

The RVU Trap (Relative Value Units): Doctors are measured and paid by RVUs — points assigned to medical activities. A 15-minute appointment: 1.5 RVUs. A 30-minute appointment: 2.3 RVUs. The math is clear: two short appointments pay better than one thorough one.

Dr. James Morrison, who left clinical practice after burnout, explains: "I could spend 30 minutes with a complex patient and earn 2.3 RVUs, or see two simple cases in that time for 3 RVUs. The system punishes thoroughness."

The Insurance Stranglehold: Insurance reimburses specific codes, not actual care. Listening isn't billable. Empathy has no code. Building relationship doesn't generate revenue. We've created a system that financially punishes good medicine.

The Scheduling Tetris: Clinics overbook assuming 20% no-shows. When everyone appears, chaos ensues. Delays cascade. Doctors rush to catch up. Patients wait hours for minutes. Everyone leaves frustrated.

The Pre-Appointment Revolution

The One-Page War Plan: I learned this after wasting dozens of appointments on disorganized rambling. Create a single page containing:

1. **Current Symptoms Hierarchy:**

- Most impactful symptom with specific examples
- Second tier symptoms with patterns
- Things that have changed since last visit
2. **The Data Dashboard:**
    - Symptom diary patterns (visualized if possible)
    - Medication responses (what helped, what hurt)
    - Triggers identified through tracking
3. **The Specific Asks:**
    - Tests you want and why
    - Referrals needed with reasoning
    - Medications to try or stop
    - Documentation needs
4. **The One Burning Question:** If everything else fails, what must be answered today?

The Research Reconnaissance:

- Google your doctor's publications — understand their interests
- Read their reviews — learn their patterns
- Check their hospital affiliations — know their resources
- Research their specialty focus — speak their language

Dr. Chen was interested in autonomic dysfunction. When I framed my POTS symptoms through that lens, suddenly I wasn't anxious — I was an interesting case.

The Support Squad Strategy: Never go alone if vulnerable. Bring someone who:

- Takes notes while you talk
- Remembers questions when you're overwhelmed
- Witnesses what's said (and not said)
- Advocates when you're too exhausted

My friend Sarah attended appointment seventeen with me. When the doctor started dismissing symptoms, she quietly said, "I've watched her collapse three times this week." External validation changed everything.

The During-Appointment Tactics

The Recording Revolution: "I have memory issues from my condition. Do you mind if I record this so I can review later?"

Watch behavior change when accountability enters. Dismissiveness becomes attentiveness. Rushed becomes thorough. Legal in single-party consent states — know your rights.

My recordings revealed patterns: Doctors who refused recording were invariably dismissive. Those who agreed were collaborative. The recording request became my screening tool.

The Strategic Interruption: When interrupted (and you will be), interrupt back: "Please let me finish — this pattern is important."

Practice this phrase. Your politeness might be killing you. One study found assertive patients received 23% more appropriate care.

The Validation Venue: Bring printed studies supporting your concerns. Not WebMD — peer-reviewed research. Highlight relevant sections. Doctors can dismiss your experience but struggle to dismiss their own literature.

I brought five studies on POTS to appointment twenty-three. The doctor who'd been skeptical suddenly became interested. Same symptoms, different framing, transformed response.

The Time Hack: "This is complex. I need a double appointment next time." Or book two consecutive slots yourself. Yes, it costs more. Your life is worth it.

The Closing Question: As they reach for the door: "What would you do if this were happening to your spouse/child?"

This question bypasses professional distance, activating personal empathy. I've seen doctors pause, return to their chair, and really think.

The Post-Appointment Protocol

The Summary Send: Email within 24 hours: "Thank you for today's appointment. To confirm my understanding:

- We discussed [symptoms]
- You recommended [treatment]
- Next steps are [specific actions]
- Questions remaining: [list]"

This creates documentation, clarifies miscommunication, and shows you're an engaged partner.

The Pattern Tracking: Document:

- What was promised vs delivered
- How you were treated
- What felt helpful or harmful
- Red flags or green lights

Patterns emerge. Doctor shopping becomes strategic selection.

The Review Reality: Leave reviews on every platform. Be specific:

- Time actually spent vs scheduled
- Listening quality
- Explanation clarity
- Respect level
- Outcome achievement

Your review might save someone else years of suffering.

The Appointment Transformation Toolkit

For Patients:

The Energy Economics Evaluation: Schedule based on your best times. If mornings are hell, book afternoons. If you crash after 2 PM, go early. Your circadian rhythm matters more than clinic convenience.

The Symptom Story Structure: "The headline is X. It started [when], feels like [specific description], happens [frequency], is triggered by [patterns noticed], affects my life by [specific impacts]."

Stories stick better than lists.

The Visual Victory: Bring graphs, charts, photos. Doctors are visual learners. My blood pressure log graph showed patterns no verbal description could convey.

The Boundary Blueprint: "I'm not comfortable with that" is a complete sentence. You can refuse treatments, request alternatives, demand dignity. Your body, your rules.

For Providers:

The First Five Revolution: Spend first five minutes just listening. No interrupting. No typing. No assuming. Just witnessing. Those five minutes save twenty later.

Dr. Amanda Roberts tried this: "Patient satisfaction increased 76%. Diagnostic accuracy improved 34%. I actually enjoyed appointments again."

The Position Power Shift: Sit at the same level as patients. Face them, not the computer. Make eye contact. Small changes, massive impact.

The Explanation Investment: Use analogies. Draw pictures. Check understanding. "Does that make sense?" isn't enough — "Can you explain back what you understood?" reveals gaps.

The Curiosity Cultivation: Replace "Have you tried therapy?" with "What have you already tried?" Assume patients are experts in their experience. They usually are.

The Systems Solutions

The Appointment Architecture Reimagined:

Tiered Time Blocks:

- 10 minutes: Simple prescription refills
- 20 minutes: Stable chronic conditions
- 30 minutes: New symptoms or complex cases

- 45 minutes: New patient or multiple conditions

Pay providers equally per time, not per patient. Quality over quantity.

The Team Approach:

- Nurse practitioner handles routine monitoring
- Physician focuses on complex decisions
- Care coordinator manages logistics
- Mental health integrated automatically

Stanford's team-based clinic: 43% better outcomes, 38% higher satisfaction, 31% lower costs.

The Technology Bridge:

- Pre-appointment questionnaires capture details
- Secure messaging between visits
- Video check-ins for simple updates
- AI scribes free doctors to focus on patients

The Patient-Reported Outcomes Integration:
Track what matters to patients:

- Function level (not just pain scale)
- Quality of life measures
- Goal achievement
- Side effect burden

When Swedish Medical Center implemented patient-reported outcomes, treatment plans improved 52%.

The Appointment Revolution Success Stories

Maria's Method: Maria, chronic migraine patient, created a appointment binder:

- One-page summary updated each visit
- Medication history with precise responses
- Trigger diary with patterns highlighted
- Questions ranked by importance
- Studies supporting requests

Result: Correct diagnosis in three appointments after three years of dismissal.

David's Documentation: David, autoimmune patient, emails summaries after every appointment, cc'ing patient advocate. Creates unignorable paper trail. Misunderstandings caught immediately. Promises tracked. Accountability established.

Result: 78% reduction in medical errors, 100% of referrals completed.

Dr. Kim's Transformation: Dr. Kim restructured her practice:

- 30-minute minimum appointments
- Patients email concerns ahead

- First ten minutes just listening
- Shared computer screen for notes
- Follow-up calls for complex cases

Result: Income maintained through quality bonuses, burnout resolved, patient outcomes improved 41%.

The Cultural Revolution Required

We need to fundamentally reimagine medical appointments:

From Transaction to Relationship: Healthcare isn't widget production. It's relationship cultivation. Every appointment builds on the last, contributing to longitudinal understanding.

From Compliance to Collaboration: Patients aren't following orders; we're co-creating solutions. Appointments become strategy sessions, not instruction deliveries.

From Time Scarcity to Time Investment: Spending 30 minutes now saves emergency visits later. Quality time prevents quantity problems.

From Provider Convenience to Patient Need: Scheduling, timing, duration, format — all should serve the person seeking help, not the system providing it.

The Metrics That Matter

Stop measuring:

- Patients seen per day
- RVUs generated
- Time per patient (as limitation)

Start measuring:

- Problems resolved first visit
- Patient understanding scores
- Shared decision achievement
- Longitudinal relationship quality
- Functional improvement
- Readmission prevention

When Cleveland Clinic changed metrics from quantity to quality, magic happened: Provider satisfaction increased, patient outcomes improved, costs actually decreased.

Your Appointment Action Plan

Before:

1. Create your one-page summary
2. Research your provider
3. Bring support if needed
4. Prepare to record
5. Plan your energy
6. Practice key phrases

During:

1. Lead with most important issue
2. Interrupt interruptions
3. Ask for clarification
4. Request appropriate time
5. Maintain boundaries
6. Get specific next steps

After:

1. Send summary email
2. Track patterns
3. Leave reviews
4. Process emotionally
5. Plan next steps
6. Share lessons learned

The Future of Medical Appointments

Imagine appointments that:

- Last as long as needed
- Build on previous conversations
- Include all relevant team members
- Happen where patients are comfortable
- Use technology to enhance, not replace
- Measure success by patient-defined outcomes
- Create healing through connection
- Transform both parties

This isn't fantasy. It's happening in pockets worldwide. Direct primary care practices. Collaborative care clinics. Patient-centered medical homes. Telemedicine innovations. The revolution is building.

The Appointment Manifesto

We declare that medical appointments should:

1. Honor the courage it takes to seek help
2. Provide time proportional to complexity
3. Build relationship alongside treatment
4. Share power between patient and provider
5. Create documentation for both parties
6. Enable questions without judgment
7. Respect boundaries and preferences
8. Measure success by life improvement
9. Generate hope alongside plans
10. Transform suffering into solution

The 15-minute appointment is not immutable law. It's a choice we've accepted too long. Every patient who demands better, every provider who practices differently, every system that measures differently — we're all part of transforming medical appointments from speed-dating with death to partnerships for life.

Your next appointment is an opportunity. Use it to model the change we need. Fifteen minutes can't contain your complexity, but it can begin your revolution.

Chapter 4: The Art of Medical Communication — When Words Become Medicine or Poison

"The difference between being heard and being healed is often just one doctor who knows how to listen with their whole body, not just their stethoscope."

The Language Barrier Nobody Admits Exists

Medical school teaches doctors to speak medicine. Life teaches patients to speak suffering. These languages share words but not meaning. "Pain" to a doctor means nociceptor activation requiring intervention. "Pain" to a patient means "I can't play with my children anymore." Same word, different universes.

I learned this during appointment number seven, describing my chest pain to a cardiologist. "Where exactly is the pain?" he asked. I pointed to my entire chest, the weight that sat there like an unwelcome cat. "Pain doesn't work that way," he declared. "Pick a specific point."

But my pain did work that way — diffuse, overwhelming, everywhere and nowhere. His inability to hear what didn't fit his framework meant seven more months without help. Words failed because translation was never attempted.

The research confirms this crisis: 40% of patients leave appointments feeling unheard. 65% of diagnostic errors stem from communication failures. We're speaking past each other while lives hang in the balance.

The Thirteen Ways Doctors Say "It's All in Your Head"

Through 2,555 days of medical encounters, I became fluent in dismissal's dialects:

1. "Have you been under stress lately?" (Translation: Your suffering is psychological)
2. "Sometimes our bodies manifest emotional pain" (Translation: You're depressed, not sick)
3. "These tests are all normal" (Translation: You're imagining things)
4. "Try yoga/meditation/mindfulness" (Translation: This isn't real medicine)

5. "You seem very focused on your symptoms" (Translation: You're obsessive)
6. "Maybe therapy would help" (Translation: See a psychiatrist, not me)
7. "Women your age often experience..." (Translation: It's hormones, hysteria's modern name)
8. "The mind-body connection is powerful" (Translation: Think yourself better)
9. "Anxiety can cause physical symptoms" (Translation: You're anxious, not ill)
10. "Let's try antidepressants" (Translation: I give up, here's Prozac)
11. "Your symptoms don't fit any pattern" (Translation: If I can't explain it, it doesn't exist)
12. "Have you considered functional disorder?" (Translation: Your body works, your mind doesn't)
13. "Quality of life is subjective" (Translation: Learn to live with it)

Each phrase landed like a small death, killing hope that this doctor, this time, might actually help. But understanding these patterns became power — I could redirect conversations before dismissal took root.

The Validation Vacuum

Here's what medical training doesn't teach: Validation isn't agreement — it's acknowledgment. You don't have to understand someone's pain to acknowledge its reality. You don't have to explain symptoms to validate their impact.

Dr. Patricia Williams changed my life with seven words: "That sounds absolutely miserable. I'm so sorry." She didn't cure me that day. She didn't even diagnose me. But she saw me, and suddenly I wasn't crazy anymore.

Studies show validation alone improves outcomes by 34%. Patients who feel heard require 38% less pain medication. Acknowledgment is literally medicine, yet it's rationed like controlled substances.

Building Your Medical Dictionary

The Translation Guide That Saved My Sanity:

Instead of: "I'm exhausted"
Say: "I'm experiencing profound fatigue that doesn't improve with rest, rating 8/10 on the fatigue severity scale"

Instead of: "I feel awful"
Say: "I'm experiencing multiple systemic symptoms

including orthostatic intolerance, post-exertional malaise, and cognitive dysfunction"

Instead of: "Something's wrong"
Say: "I've noticed a pattern of symptoms that correlate with [specific triggers] and significantly impact my activities of daily living"

Instead of: "You have to help me"
Say: "I need diagnostic clarity and a treatment plan that addresses these specific functional limitations"

Instead of: "Nothing works"
Say: "I've tried X, Y, and Z with these specific results [bring documentation]. What alternatives would you recommend?"

The key isn't becoming emotionless — it's translating emotion into language medicine recognizes.

The Power Dynamics Embedded in Every Word

Medical language maintains hierarchy. "Compliance" means obedience. "Non-compliant" means bad patient. "Drug-seeking" means unworthy of pain relief. "Difficult patient" means someone who asks questions.

I was labeled "non-compliant" for refusing a medication that had previously caused severe side effects. The label followed me through referrals, prejudicing each new doctor. When I finally accessed my records, I found "anxious," "difficult," and "possibly somatizing" scattered like landmines through my chart.

Language in medical records becomes verdict without trial. One doctor's "seems anxious" becomes another's justification for dismissal. The pen isn't just mightier than the sword — in medicine, it is the sword.

The Strategic Conversation Architecture

The Opening Gambit:
"Thank you for seeing me. I've prepared a brief summary of my symptoms and their impact. I have three specific questions I'm hoping we can address today."

This establishes you as organized partner, not chaotic patient. It sets agenda, shows respect for time, demonstrates preparation.

The Evidence Escalator:
Level 1: Personal observation ("I've noticed...")
Level 2: Documented patterns ("My symptom diary shows...")
Level 3: External validation ("My partner has observed...")

Level 4: Medical literature ("Studies indicate...")
Level 5: Previous medical documentation ("As Dr. X noted...")

Start at Level 1. Escalate only as needed. Meeting resistance with increasing evidence rather than emotion maintains professional dynamic.

The Redirect Response:
When conversation veers toward dismissal:
"I understand that perspective. However, I'm experiencing measurable physical symptoms that need addressing. Can we focus on those?"

Acknowledge their position, assert your reality, redirect to actionable discussion.

The Clarification Checkpoint:
"Let me make sure I understand correctly. You're saying [repeat back]. Is that accurate?"

This prevents misunderstanding, creates documentation opportunity, forces clear communication.

The Commitment Close:
"So our plan is [specific actions]. You'll [their commitments]. I'll [your commitments]. We'll reassess in [timeframe]. Should I schedule that follow-up now?"

Specificity prevents promises from evaporating.

The Witnessing Revolution

Bring a witness. Always. Their presence changes dynamics entirely. Doctors perform differently with audiences. Dismissiveness decreases 67% with witnesses present. Documentation improves 45%. Respect increases measurably.

Sarah, my appointment companion, developed a system: She took notes silently unless I gave our predetermined signal (touching my ear). Then she'd interject with observations: "I've noticed her symptoms are worst in mornings," or "The pattern seems cyclical, about every 28 days."

External validation carries weight internal experience doesn't. It shouldn't be necessary, but it's effective.

The Documentation Dialectic

The Real-Time Record:
During appointments, repeat and record:
"So you're saying the test results rule out cardiac involvement?"
"You're recommending I try this medication for three months?"
"You don't think further testing is necessary?"

This creates immediate accountability, prevents later denial, clarifies in moment.

The Paper Trail Power:
Email after every appointment:
"Dear Dr. [Name], Thank you for today's appointment. To confirm our discussion..."

CC yourself, blind CC patient advocate if you have one. Paper trails prevent gaslighting, create legal record, ensure accountability.

The Chart Challenge:
Request your records regularly. Challenge inaccuracies immediately:
"The record states I declined treatment. Actually, I declined that specific medication due to documented adverse reaction, but requested alternatives."

Fighting for accurate records is fighting for your future care.

The Emotional Labor Economics

Medical communication requires enormous emotional labor from patients. We must:

- Remain calm while discussing terrifying symptoms
- Stay rational when feeling dismissed
- Be assertive without seeming aggressive
- Educate without condescending

- Advocate without alienating

This labor is unpaid, unrecognized, but absolutely essential. I spent approximately 500 hours learning to communicate effectively with medical providers — time that should've been spent healing.

The unfair truth: Sick people must work hardest to be heard.

Communication Innovations That Actually Work

The Teach-Back Method:
Progressive clinics now use "teach-back" — patients explain understanding before leaving. Comprehension increases 73%, errors decrease 49%.

The Open Notes Movement:
Institutions sharing notes with patients immediately see communication improve. Patients catch errors, provide context, feel included. Trust increases, lawsuits decrease.

The Narrative Medicine Approach:
Columbia's Narrative Medicine program teaches doctors to hear stories, not just symptoms. Graduates show 45% better diagnostic accuracy, 62% higher patient satisfaction.

The Shared Decision Making Model:
When patients and providers decide together, adherence improves 68%, regret decreases 54%, outcomes improve across all metrics.

The Cultural Context Complications

Medical communication assumes shared cultural context that doesn't exist. When my grandmother, Holocaust survivor, said "I'm fine," she meant "I'm not actively dying." When doctors heard "fine," they heard "no intervention needed."

Cultural translation requires:

- *Understanding what silence means in different cultures*
- *Recognizing how pain is expressed differently*
- *Knowing when directness offends or empowers*
- *Adapting to different concepts of body and illness*

Medicine pretends to be objective, but communication is inherently cultural. Ignoring this kills people.

The Gender Dynamics Destroying Communication

Women's symptoms are minimized 73% more than men's. We're interrupted more, believed less, offered psychological explanations more frequently. Our pain requires more evidence to be treated equally.

I learned to bring my husband to appointments. Not for support — for credibility. When he repeated exactly what I'd said, suddenly it became valid. The same words, different gender, transformed response.

This isn't about individual sexist doctors — it's about systematic bias embedded in medical communication patterns.

The Technology Bridge and Barrier

Telemedicine revealed communication truths:

- Without physical presence, words matter more
- Screen fatigue affects both parties
- Technology can enhance or inhibit connection
- Digital divide affects care access

But also opportunities:

- Recording capabilities for review
- Chat functions for clarification
- Screen sharing for education
- Asynchronous communication for complex cases

My best medical communication happened over video — doctor couldn't physically leave, had to listen fully.

The Script Library That Saves Lives

For Seeking Second Opinions:
"I value your expertise and want to make fully informed decisions. I'm seeking additional perspectives to ensure I understand all options."

For Refusing Treatment:
"I've carefully considered this treatment. Based on my previous experiences and current circumstances, I'm declining at this time. What alternatives would you suggest?"

For Demanding Referrals:
"Given the complexity and persistence of these symptoms, I need specialist evaluation. Which specialist would you recommend?"

For Challenging Dismissal:
"I understand you don't have answers currently. However, these symptoms are significantly impacting my life. What investigative steps can we take?"

For Requesting Time:
"This is complex and important. I need time to process this information. Can we schedule a follow-up to discuss questions that arise?"

The Nonverbal Vocabulary

55% of communication is body language, 38% is tone, only 7% is words. In medical encounters:

- Maintain eye contact (shows engagement, demands attention)
- Sit straight (indicates seriousness, prevents dismissal)
- Take notes (demonstrates investment, creates accountability)
- Pause after speaking (forces response, prevents interruption)
- Mirror their posture (builds unconscious rapport)

When doctors turned away from me toward computers, I'd pause mid-sentence. The silence pulled them back. Attention must be demanded, not hoped for.

The Communication Revolution Manifesto

We demand medical communication that:

1. **Assumes competence** — Patients understand more than you think
2. **Shares power** — Dialogue, not monologue
3. **Validates experience** — Acknowledgment before explanation
4. **Invites questions** — Without judgment or time pressure
5. **Admits uncertainty** — "I don't know" is acceptable
6. **Respects boundaries** — "No" is complete sentence
7. **Provides translation** — Medical terms explained clearly
8. **Ensures understanding** — Confirmation before conclusion
9. **Documents accurately** — Records reflect reality
10. **Builds relationship** — Connection enables healing

The Stories That Transform

Marcus, chronic pain patient, created communication cards: "I need a moment," "Please speak slower," "I need to see that written." Simple tools that transformed his care.

Dr. Jennifer Lee posts appointment prep sheets online: "What to bring," "How to describe symptoms," "Questions to ask." Empowering patients before they arrive.

Trinity Medical Center trained all staff in "compassionate communication." Patient satisfaction increased 84%, medical errors decreased 43%, staff burnout reduced 38%.

Your Communication Action Plan

Before Appointments:

- Write out key points
- Practice difficult phrases
- Prepare evidence hierarchy
- Plan emotional regulation
- Arrange witness

During Encounters:

- Lead with clear summary
- Use medical terminology
- Document in real-time
- Redirect dismissal
- Confirm understanding

After Interactions:

- Send summary email
- Update your records
- Process emotions
- Share lessons learned
- Plan improvements

For Providers:

- Listen without interrupting
- Validate before explaining
- Admit uncertainty
- Share decision-making
- Document collaboratively

The Future We're Speaking Into Existence

Imagine medical communication where:

- Patients' words carry equal weight
- Providers listen with curiosity
- Translation happens automatically
- Understanding is verified
- Stories inform treatment
- Silence has space
- Questions are welcomed
- Answers are honest
- Uncertainty is acceptable
- Connection enables healing

This future requires all of us to change how we speak and listen. Every conversation is opportunity for revolution. Every word can heal or harm. Every interaction builds the system we need.

The revolution doesn't shout — it speaks clearly, listens deeply, translates constantly, and refuses to accept that miscommunication is inevitable.

Your voice matters. Your words have power. Your story deserves to be heard. And if they won't listen, speak louder, clearer, and bring witnesses.

The conversation that saves your life might be the next one. Make it count.

Chapter 5: Diagnostic Odysseys — When Finding Answers Becomes a Full-Time Job Without Pay

"The cruelest part of diagnostic purgatory isn't the not knowing — it's everyone else's certainty that if it hasn't been found, it doesn't exist."

The Seven-Year Education in Medical Mystery

2,555 days. That's how long my body posed questions medicine couldn't answer. Each day teaching me that diagnosis isn't discovery — it's archaeology, slowly brushing dust from buried truth, hoping the fragments form a picture before you run out of time, money, or will to continue.

The average rare disease patient sees 16 doctors over 7.6 years before diagnosis. I hit those numbers precisely, like my body was following some cosmic curriculum in medical frustration. But those statistics don't capture the texture of those years — the 3 AM googling, the medical journal rabbit holes, the support group scrolling, the desperate hope that this doctor, this test, this theory might finally explain why standing up became impossible.

Day 1: "It's probably just stress"
Day 90: "Have you tried yoga?"
Day 365: "All your tests are normal"
Day 730: "Maybe it's psychological"
Day 1,095: "You're too young for anything serious"
Day 1,460: "Sometimes we never find answers"
Day 1,825: "Have you considered this might be anxiety?"
Day 2,190: "Let me refer you to psychiatry"
Day 2,555: "Have you heard of POTS?"

One question. Three letters. Seven years.

The Diagnostic Industrial Complex

Healthcare loves acute problems. Heart attack? We've got protocols. Broken bone? Clear pathway. Infection? Treatment algorithm. But chronic, complex, multi-system conditions? We might as well be asking medicine to solve poetry with mathematics.

The system is designed for diagnostic efficiency, not accuracy:

- *Average primary care visit: 15 minutes*
- *Average time to interruption: 11 seconds*
- *Tests ordered to avoid lawsuits: 47%*
- *Referrals made to pass problems along: 63%*

We've built a diagnostic assembly line for problems that require artisan attention.

The Test Trap Paradox

"Your tests are normal" might be medicine's most violent phrase. It sounds like good news but lands like gaslighting. Normal tests don't mean normal life. They mean your suffering doesn't fit our measurements.

My normal tests:

- *14 complete blood counts (perfect)*
- *8 EKGs (textbook)*
- *3 echocardiograms (beautiful heart)*
- *2 stress tests (passed with flying colors)*
- *1 cardiac MRI (structurally sound)*
- *4 chest X-rays (clear)*
- *2 CT scans (unremarkable)*
- *Countless other tests (all normal)*

Total cost: $73,000
Diagnostic value: Zero

But here's the revolution: I started requesting different tests. Not more tests — different ones. Orthostatic vitals. Tilt table test. Autonomic function studies. Tests that measured what I was experiencing, not what doctors assumed I should be experiencing.

The tilt table test that finally diagnosed POTS cost 1,200. Seven years and 1,200. Seven years and 73,000 in wrong tests, versus one right test that insurance initially denied as "experimental."

The Pattern Recognition University

Patients become pattern recognition machines. We have to. Doctors see snapshots; we live the movie. We notice:

- *The Tuesday migraines*
- *The post-meal crashes*
- *The weather correlations*
- *The menstrual cycle connections*
- *The stress response delays*
- *The exercise aftermath*
- *The sleep position effects*

I tracked everything in spreadsheets that would make data scientists weep. Heart rate, blood pressure, temperature, symptoms, food, weather, stress, sleep, activity. Patterns emerged that no 15-minute appointment could capture:

- *Heart rate increased 40+ BPM upon standing (POTS signature)*
- *Symptoms worse in heat (autonomic dysfunction)*
- *Improvement with salt/fluids (blood volume issue)*
- *Crashes 24-48 hours after exertion (post-exertional malaise)*

When I presented these patterns to doctor number 33, she didn't dismiss them. She said, "You've already diagnosed yourself. Let's confirm it."

The Differential Diagnosis Your Doctor Won't Consider

Medical training teaches doctors to think horses when they hear hoofbeats. But some of us are zebras. And medicine is terrible at recognizing stripes.

Common conditions doctors miss:

- POTS (Postural Orthostatic Tachycardia Syndrome): Affects 3 million Americans, average diagnosis time 6 years
- EDS (Ehlers-Danlos Syndrome): 1 in 5,000 people, usually dismissed as "being flexible"
- MCAS (Mast Cell Activation Syndrome): Unknown prevalence, mistaken for allergies or anxiety
- Autoimmune conditions: Women wait average 4.6 years for diagnosis
- Endometriosis: 7-12 years to diagnosis despite affecting 10% of women
- Fibromyalgia: Often dismissed entirely despite affecting 4 million Americans

These aren't rare. They're rarely diagnosed.

The Gender Gap That Kills

Women wait longer for diagnosis, receive more psychological explanations, get less pain medication, and die more from medical dismissal.

The numbers are damning:

- Women 50% more likely to be misdiagnosed after heart attack
- Women wait 65 minutes in emergency rooms versus men's 49 minutes
- Women's pain dismissed as emotional 83% of initial presentations
- Autoimmune diseases affect women 75% more but research funding is 30% less

I learned to bring male witnesses to appointments. When my husband described my symptoms, suddenly they became real. Same symptoms, different gender describing them, diagnosis achieved. The misogyny is systemic, embedded in diagnostic algorithms that default male.

The Specialist Spiral

Primary care to cardiology to neurology to rheumatology to psychiatry back to primary care. Each specialist examining their organ system, nobody seeing the human.

The referral notes read like medical hot potato:

- "Please evaluate for cardiac cause" (It's not cardiac)
- "Please assess for neurological etiology" (It's not neurological)
- "Please rule out rheumatological condition" (It's not rheumatological)
- "Please consider psychological factors" (It's not psychological)

Meanwhile, the patient deteriorates while being shuffled between departments that don't communicate except through notes that say nothing.

The Insurance Obstacle Course

Insurance companies practice medicine without licenses. They decide which tests you can have, which specialists you can see, which treatments you can try. They're not interested in diagnosis — they're interested in denial.

My insurance battles:

- Tilt table test denied as "experimental" (It's been standard since 1986)
- Specialist referral denied as "not medically necessary" (I couldn't stand up)
- Genetic testing denied as "investigational" (It would have saved years)

- Treatment denied as "off-label" (Most treatments are off-label)

Each denial required appeals, documentation, physician letters, and hours on hold. I became a professional insurance fighter because the alternative was dying undiagnosed.

The Dr. Google Phenomenon

"Don't Google your symptoms" is advice given by people who've never been medically abandoned. When medicine fails you, the Internet becomes your medical school.

Yes, cyberchondria is real. But so is cyberdiagnosis. Patients online diagnosed my POTS two years before doctors did. Support groups provided treatment strategies that worked. Medical Twitter taught me more than most appointments.

The key is curation:

- Peer-reviewed journals (PubMed, not Pinterest)
- Reputable medical sites (Mayo Clinic, not random blogs)
- Patient organizations (vetted information)
- Support groups (pattern recognition)
- Medical Twitter (actual doctors discussing cases)

I printed studies, highlighted relevant sections, brought them to appointments. Some doctors were offended. The good ones were intrigued.

The Diagnostic Activism Toolkit

The Symptom Diary That Delivers:

- Date/time stamps for everything
- Severity scales (1-10) for consistency
- Trigger identification
- Pattern highlighting
- Photo documentation when visible
- Witness statements when available

The Test Request Strategy:
"Based on my symptoms and research, I believe [specific test] could provide diagnostic clarity. Can we discuss this?"

Not: "I want this test"
But: "Let's explore whether this test makes sense"

The Referral Request Script:
"Given the complexity and persistence of these symptoms, I think specialist evaluation is warranted. Would you recommend [specific specialty] or suggest another direction?"

The Second Opinion Approach:
"I value your expertise and want to make fully

informed decisions. I'm seeking additional perspectives to ensure we're not missing anything."

The Insurance Appeal Arsenal:

- Letter of medical necessity from doctor
- Peer-reviewed studies supporting test/treatment
- Documentation of failed alternatives
- Personal impact statement
- Timeline of diagnostic journey
- Cost comparison (test now vs. emergency care later)

The Alternative Investigation Avenues

When traditional medicine fails, patients get creative:

Direct-to-Consumer Testing:

- Genetic testing (revealed my EDS)
- Microbiome analysis (identified gut issues)
- Hormone panels (found imbalances)
- Food sensitivity testing (discovered triggers)

Not all are valid, but some provide clues medicine missed.

Clinical Trials:
Sometimes being a research subject provides better care than being a patient. Clinical trials offer:

- Cutting-edge treatments
- Intensive monitoring
- Motivated providers
- Free care

Functional Medicine:
Expensive, often not covered, but sometimes finds what conventional medicine misses:

- Comprehensive testing
- Systems approach
- Root cause investigation
- Time to actually listen

Medical Tourism:
Other countries sometimes diagnose what America misses:

- Different diagnostic approaches
- Tests unavailable in US
- Specialists in specific conditions
- Often cheaper even with travel

The Psychological Toll Nobody Measures

Diagnostic uncertainty creates unique psychological torture:

- Imposter syndrome (maybe I am imagining it)
- Medical trauma (from repeated dismissal)
- Anticipatory grief (for the life you're losing)
- Relationship strain (being believed is exhausting)
- Identity crisis (who am I if not diagnosed?)
- Decision fatigue (from constant self-advocacy)

I spent $15,000 on therapy to survive the diagnosis journey. Mental health support should be standard during diagnostic odysseys, not luxury.

The Diagnosis Day That Changes Everything and Nothing

When Dr. Chen said "You have POTS," I cried for three hours. Not from sadness — from validation. Seven years of being told nothing was wrong, and suddenly I had three letters that explained everything.

But diagnosis isn't cure. It's explanation. It's validation. It's direction. But it's also beginning, not ending.

The average POTS patient improves 60% with treatment. But getting that treatment required:

- Finding doctors who knew POTS
- Convincing insurance to cover treatment
- Trial and error with medications
- Lifestyle overhaul
- Continued advocacy
- Accepting chronic as permanent resident

Diagnosis is like getting a map after being lost for years. Helpful, essential, but you still have to walk the path.

The Systemic Solutions Required

Diagnostic Centers of Excellence:
Specialized centers for complex cases where:

- Multiple specialists collaborate
- Time isn't constrained
- Testing is comprehensive
- Patterns are investigated
- Patients are believed

AI-Assisted Pattern Recognition:
Computers excel at pattern recognition. Feed them symptoms, tests, history — find connections humans miss.

Patient-Reported Outcome Integration:
What matters to patients should drive diagnostic investigation, not what's easy to test.

Diagnostic Justice Initiatives:

- Reduced diagnostic disparities
- Cultural competence in diagnosis
- Gender bias training
- Rare disease education
- Complex case protocols

Time Banking for Diagnosis:
Allowing longer appointments for complex cases without financial penalty to providers.

The Diagnostic Revolution Already Beginning

At Stanford, patients with mysterious symptoms enter diagnostic programs where teams spend weeks investigating. Diagnosis rate: 78%.

In the Netherlands, diagnostic detectives take on cold cases. Success rate: 63%.

The Undiagnosed Diseases Network connects patients with research teams. 35% get answers.

CrowdMed lets medical professionals worldwide review cases. 60% receive helpful insights.

These aren't miracles — they're what happens when diagnosis gets appropriate resources.

Your Diagnostic Battle Plan

Year 1: Foundation Building

- *Document everything*
- *Track patterns obsessively*
- *Build medical team*
- *Join support groups*
- *Start researching*

Year 2: Pattern Recognition

- *Identify triggers*
- *Map symptom cycles*
- *Correlate with life factors*
- *Present patterns to doctors*
- *Request specific tests*

Year 3: Strategic Escalation

- *Seek specialists*
- *Request referrals*
- *Consider second opinions*
- *Explore alternative testing*
- *Document insurance denials*

Year 4+: Creative Solutions

- *Direct-to-consumer testing*
- *Functional medicine*
- *Clinical trials*
- *Medical tourism*
- *Diagnostic programs*

Throughout: Psychological Support

- *Therapy for medical trauma*
- *Support groups for validation*
- *Boundaries with doubters*
- *Self-compassion practice*
- *Hope maintenance*

The Diagnosis Manifesto

We demand diagnostic justice:

1. **Time proportional to complexity** — *Complex cases need more than 15 minutes*
2. **Pattern recognition over snapshot assessment** — *Longitudinal view matters*
3. **Patient expertise integration** — *We know our bodies*
4. **Saying "I don't know" instead of "it's psychological"** — *Uncertainty isn't psychiatric*
5. **Collaborative investigation** — *Partners, not subjects*
6. **Insurance coverage for diagnostic journeys** — *Not just confirmed conditions*
7. **Mental health support during uncertainty** — *Diagnostic trauma is real*
8. **Cultural and gender competence** — *Bias kills*
9. **Rare disease education** — *Zebras exist*
10. **Hope without false promises** — *Honesty with compassion*

The Truth About Diagnostic Odysseys

They're not journeys — they're wars. Wars against disbelief, dismissal, debt, despair. Wars fought while sick, without training, against systems designed for simplicity.

But we're winning. Every patient who persists, every doctor who listens, every diagnosis achieved after years of searching — these are victories that change the landscape for those behind us.

My seven years weren't wasted. They were education. In persistence. In pattern recognition. In self-advocacy. In system navigation. In maintaining hope when experts offer none.

Your diagnostic odyssey is valid whether it takes months or decades. Your persistence isn't pathological — it's powerful. Your research isn't obsessive — it's necessary. Your knowing isn't anxiety — it's expertise.

The diagnosis you seek exists. The answer is out there. And sometimes, you'll have to become your own diagnostic detective to find it.

The revolution happens when we stop accepting "we don't know" as ending and start seeing it as beginning. When we recognize that patients and providers together solve what neither can alone.

Keep searching. Keep documenting. Keep pushing. Keep hoping.

Your diagnosis is coming. And when it does, you'll use everything you learned getting there to help others still searching.

That's how diagnostic odysseys become diagnostic revolutions.

Chapter 6: Treatment Trials and Errors — The Human Guinea Pig Chronicles

"Every patient becomes a scientist, running experiments on a sample size of one, where the subject is yourself and failure isn't just data — it's your life falling apart."

The Treatment Lottery Nobody Wins

The moment after diagnosis should feel like victory. Finally, answers. Finally, treatment. Finally, hope. Instead, it's the starting gun for a different race —

one where the finish line keeps moving and the track is littered with side effects, false starts, and insurance denials.

My POTS diagnosis came with a treatment "menu" that read like pharmaceutical poetry:

- Beta blockers (made me bradycardic)
- Fludrocortisone (hello, potassium depletion)
- Midodrine (supine hypertension, anyone?)
- Pyridostigmine (gastrointestinal rebellion)
- Ivabradine (not FDA approved, good luck with insurance)
- Salt tablets (8 grams daily, yes really)
- Compression garments (medical spanx in summer heat)
- Exercise protocol (when standing is optional?)

Seven years seeking diagnosis. Three more years finding treatment that worked. A decade of my life as clinical trial with no control group, no ethical oversight, and no hazard pay.

The First-Line Failure Phenomenon

Medicine has protocols. First-line treatments, second-line, third-line — as if illness follows corporate hierarchy. But what happens when first-line fails? When second-line makes you sicker? When third-line isn't covered by insurance?

You become what I call a "treatment refugee" — someone who's tried everything recommended and now lives in the wasteland beyond protocols.

Statistics they don't advertise:

- First-line treatments fail in 40-60% of chronic illness patients
- Average patient tries 5-7 medications before finding relief
- 30% never find adequate treatment
- 67% experience significant side effects
- 45% stop treatment due to side effects worse than symptoms

The dirty secret: Most treatments weren't tested on people like us. Clinical trials exclude complex patients, elderly people, women of childbearing age, people with multiple conditions. The treatments are tested on the healthiest sick people, then prescribed to the sickest sick people.

The Side Effect Roulette

Every medication comes with a novel-length list of potential side effects that reads like a sadistic creative writing exercise. "May cause drowsiness" sounds manageable until you're sleeping 18 hours and still exhausted. "Mild nausea" becomes "can't keep water down." "Temporary adjustment period" stretches into months of misery.

My side effect greatest hits:

- Beta blocker: Heart rate so low I couldn't climb stairs
- SSRI (for "anxiety"): Serotonin syndrome that landed me in ER
- Gabapentin: Cognitive fog that stole my words
- Prednisone: Mood swings that destroyed relationships
- Muscle relaxants: Weakness that required wheelchair
- Tramadol: Withdrawal that felt like dying
- Birth control (for "hormone regulation"): Stroke-level migraines

Each medication a hope that became harm. Each trial an investment of weeks or months to know if it helped, hurt, or did nothing. Each failure requiring careful weaning to avoid withdrawal while simultaneously starting the next experiment.

The Insurance Authorization Theatre

Insurance companies practice medicine without licenses, deciding which treatments you can try based on cost, not clinical need. The authorization process is deliberately exhausting, hoping you'll give up before they have to pay.

The typical authorization dance:

1. Doctor prescribes medication
2. Pharmacy says insurance denied
3. Insurance demands "prior authorization"
4. Doctor submits paperwork
5. Insurance denies as "not medically necessary"
6. Doctor appeals with more documentation
7. Insurance demands you fail cheaper alternatives first
8. You spend months on medications that don't work
9. Document failure meticulously
10. Insurance maybe approves original medication
11. Copay is still unaffordable
12. You ration or go without

I spent approximately 300 hours fighting insurance for treatments my doctors deemed necessary. That's 7.5 work weeks of unpaid labor while sick, fighting for the right to try to get better.

The Off-Label Underground

Most treatments for complex conditions are "off-label" — medications approved for one thing, used for another. Insurance loves denying these.

But off-label use isn't experimental — it's how medicine evolves.

Off-label treatments that saved me:

- Propranolol (for migraines, used for POTS)
- Low-dose naltrexone (for pain, used for immune modulation)
- Ketamine (anesthetic, used for chronic pain)
- Modafinil (for narcolepsy, used for fatigue)

Getting these required:

- Finding doctors willing to prescribe off-label
- Extensive documentation of medical necessity
- Often paying out of pocket
- Sometimes ordering from other countries
- Always accepting legal and medical risk

The off-label underground is where desperate patients become amateur pharmacologists, sharing what works in support groups because medical literature hasn't caught up to lived experience.

The Lifestyle Prescription Paradox

"Just exercise more!" they say to someone who faints standing up.
"Reduce stress!" they suggest while you're fighting insurance, missing work, and losing relationships.

"Eat better!" they recommend when medical costs leave food budget decimated.
"Get more sleep!" they advise when symptoms and medication side effects destroy rest.

Lifestyle modifications are prescribed like they're free and easy. They're neither.

My "lifestyle modification" reality:

- Exercise program: $200/month specialized physical therapy
- Stress reduction: $150/session therapy not covered by insurance
- Dietary changes: $500/month for specific foods
- Sleep improvement: 2000forstudies,2000forstudies,5000 for CPAP
- Compression garments: $300 each, need multiple
- Cooling vest for heat intolerance: $400
- Shower chair to prevent fainting: $150
- Heart rate monitor: $300
- Blood pressure cuff: $100

Total "lifestyle" cost: Over $15,000 annually. That's not lifestyle — that's luxury most can't afford.

The Alternative Medicine Money Pit

When conventional medicine fails, desperation drives us to alternatives. The alternative medicine industry generates $82 billion annually from people failed by traditional healthcare.

My expensive experiments:

- Acupuncture: 100/session,twiceweekly(100/session,twice weekly(800/month)
- Naturopathy: 300consultation,300consultation,200/month supplements
- Functional medicine: $500 consultation, not covered
- Chiropractic: $75/adjustment, three times weekly
- Reiki: $100/session (expensive placebo)
- Infrared sauna: $50/session
- Cryotherapy: $65/session
- Float tanks: $80/session
- CBD oil: $200/month
- Supplements: $300/month for the "protocol"

Total spent on alternatives: 30,000overthreeyearsTotalthatactuallyhelped:Maybe30,000overthreeyearsTotalthatactuallyhelped:Maybe3,000 worth

Not all alternative medicine is scam, but vulnerability makes us perfect marks for those selling hope in bottles.

The Treatment Activism Toolkit

The Treatment Spreadsheet:
Track everything:

- Medication name, dose, dates
- Side effects with severity ratings
- Effectiveness for each symptom
- Interactions discovered
- Cost per month
- Insurance battles required
- Quality of life impact (-10 to +10)

This becomes your evidence for what works, what doesn't, and why you won't try something again.

The Titration Protocol:
Start lower than recommended, increase slower than suggested. Most protocols assume robust bodies. Sensitive systems need gentler approaches.

My rule: Start at 1/4 recommended dose, increase by 1/4 every two weeks, stop when helping or harming becomes clear.

The Side Effect Negotiation:
"The side effects are intolerable" is valid reason to stop treatment.
"I need to try something else" is complete explanation.

"Quality of life matters more than lab values" is your right.

The Insurance Appeal Arsenal:

- Letter of medical necessity (detailed, with references)
- Peer-reviewed studies supporting off-label use
- Documentation of failed alternatives
- Cost analysis (medication vs. hospitalization)
- Personal impact statement
- Provider peer-to-peer review request

The Treatment Contract:
With your doctor, establish:

- Trial period for each treatment
- Specific outcomes to measure
- Side effect thresholds for stopping
- Check-in schedule
- Exit strategy if failing

The Compound Pharmacy Revolution

Commercial medications assume average bodies. Compound pharmacies create customized solutions.

Game-changers from compounding:

- Medications without problematic fillers
- Doses between commercial strengths
- Combination preparations
- Alternative delivery methods
- Discontinued medications recreated

Yes, it's often more expensive and not covered. But when you're allergic to corn and every pill contains corn starch, compounding becomes survival.

The Clinical Trial Calculation

Sometimes being a research subject provides better care than being a patient.

Clinical trial benefits:

- Free medication
- Intensive monitoring
- Motivated providers
- Cutting-edge treatments
- Contributing to science

Clinical trial risks:

- Placebo possibility
- Unknown side effects
- Rigid protocols
- Travel requirements
- Time commitment

I participated in three trials. One helped immensely, one did nothing, one made me sicker. Still better odds than standard treatment roulette.

The International Treatment Tourism

Other countries have treatments America doesn't. Sometimes medical tourism makes sense.

Treatments available elsewhere:

- Stem cell therapy (Mexico, Panama)
- Hyperbaric oxygen (more accessible abroad)
- Medications not FDA approved
- Procedures insurance won't cover
- Specialists in rare conditions

The calculation: $10,000 for treatment abroad versus years of suffering awaiting American approval.

The Shared Decision-Making Myth

"Shared decision-making" sounds collaborative. In reality, it's often doctors presenting options they prefer, patients choosing from limited menus, insurance determining final say.

True shared decision-making requires:

- Full disclosure of all options
- Honest discussion of uncertainties
- Patient values driving choices
- Risk tolerance assessment
- Quality of life prioritization
- Financial reality consideration

This happened once in ten years. Dr. Martinez said, "Here are six options. Let's discuss what matters most to you and design a plan." Revolutionary.

The Treatment Success Redefinition

Medical success: Lab values normalize
Patient success: Can shower without fainting

Medical success: Disease markers improve
Patient success: Can work part-time

Medical success: Symptoms reduce 30%
Patient success: Can play with children

We need new metrics that measure what matters to patients, not just what's easy to measure.

The Peer Treatment Intelligence Network

Patients share treatment intelligence with military precision:

Facebook groups: "Has anyone tried X for Y?"
Reddit threads: Detailed treatment experiences
Twitter: Real-time side effect reporting
Discord servers: 24/7 support during treatment trials
Spreadsheets: Crowdsourced effectiveness data

This peer network provides information no clinical trial captures — real-world effectiveness in complex patients.

The Treatment Trauma Nobody Discusses

Every failed treatment is grief. Every side effect is betrayal. Every insurance denial is abandonment. Treatment trauma compounds illness trauma.

The psychological toll:

- Hope exhaustion from repeated failure
- Medical PTSD from adverse reactions
- Decision paralysis from too many failures
- Relationship strain from mood effects
- Identity crisis from cognitive changes
- Anxiety about trying anything new

I needed therapy specifically for treatment trauma. The illness was hard enough; the treatment journey nearly broke me.

The Polypharmacy Puzzle

Multiple conditions mean multiple medications mean multiple interactions nobody fully understands.

My peak medication load:

- 8 prescription medications
- 12 supplements
- 4 as-needed medications
- 3 topical treatments

That's 27 substances interacting in ways no study has examined. Each prescriber focused on their specialty, nobody managing the whole. I became my own interaction checker, my own pharmacist, my own adverse event monitor.

The Treatment Revolution Required

Personalized Medicine Reality:

- Genetic testing for medication metabolism
- Biomarker-driven treatment selection
- Individual response prediction

- Customized dosing protocols
- Real-world evidence integration

Treatment Decision Support:

- AI-assisted interaction checking
- Patient-reported outcome integration
- Predictive modeling for success
- Side effect likelihood calculation
- Cost-effectiveness analysis

Insurance Reform:

- Off-label coverage when indicated
- Alternative treatment inclusion
- Failed treatment acknowledgment
- Faster authorization process
- Patient experience consideration

Provider Education:

- Complex patient management
- Polypharmacy navigation
- Side effect sensitivity
- Quality of life prioritization
- Shared decision reality

Your Treatment Navigation Strategy

Before Starting Treatment:

1. Research extensively (medical literature, patient experiences)
2. Document baseline symptoms
3. Clarify success metrics
4. Establish stop criteria
5. Plan for side effects
6. Ensure support system
7. Calculate true costs

During Treatment:

1. Track everything obsessively
2. Communicate changes immediately
3. Don't suffer in silence
4. Advocate for adjustments
5. Connect with others on same treatment
6. Monitor interactions
7. Trust your body's wisdom

When Treatment Fails:

1. Document why it failed
2. Allow grief time
3. Analyze lessons learned
4. Share experience with others
5. Request different approach
6. Consider alternatives
7. Maintain hope

The Treatment Manifesto

We demand treatment approaches that:

1. **Acknowledge individual variation** — One size fits none
2. **Prioritize quality of life** — Living matters more than labs
3. **Include patient expertise** — We know our bodies
4. **Provide honest information** — Uncertainties included
5. **Enable true choice** — All options, not just preferred
6. **Support failed attempts** — Without blame or shame
7. **Consider financial reality** — Bankruptcy isn't healing
8. **Integrate peer experience** — Collective wisdom matters
9. **Measure patient-defined success** — Our goals, not yours
10. **Treat humans, not conditions** — Whole person, whole life

The Truth About Treatment

Treatment is experiment. Every medication is hypothesis. Every intervention is theory. We're all running personal clinical trials with no control group, no safety board, and no compensation for our contribution to medical knowledge.

But we persist because the alternative is accepting unnecessary suffering. We become scientists of our own bodies, researchers of our own conditions, advocates for our own care.

My treatment journey cost me:

- $75,000 in direct costs
- 1,000+ hours in management
- Relationships strained by side effects
- Career derailed by cognitive impacts
- Dreams deferred by energy depletion

But it also taught me:

- Persistence pays
- Patient expertise is real
- Small improvements compound
- Community provides answers medicine doesn't
- Hope survives repeated disappointment
- Healing happens in unexpected ways

Your treatment journey is valid whether you find perfect solution or acceptable compromise. Your experiments matter whether they succeed or fail. Your expertise grows with every trial.

The revolution happens when we stop accepting treatment as something done to us and start demanding treatment done with us. When we recognize that patients hold essential data about what works in real bodies living real lives.

Keep trying. Keep tracking. Keep sharing. Keep hoping.

Your treatment is out there. And when you find what works, you'll light the path for others still searching.

That's how treatment trials become treatment triumphs.

Chapter 7: The Insurance Battle — Fighting for Care in a System Designed for Denial

"Insurance companies have perfected the art of collecting premiums while denying care, creating a system where being insured doesn't mean being covered, and being covered doesn't mean being treated."

The Great American Healthcare Illusion

I have "good" insurance. Employer-sponsored. "Platinum" level. 800monthlypremium.800monthlypremium.2,000 deductible. 20% coinsurance. $8,000 out-of-pocket maximum. These numbers meant safety until I got sick and learned that insurance is less safety net and more spider web — designed to trap, not catch.

Year one of illness: Hit out-of-pocket maximum by March
Year two: Maximum by February
Year three through seven: Maximum by January 15th

That's $56,000 in seven years WITH "good" insurance. The uninsured aren't the only ones going bankrupt from medical bills — the insured are drowning too, just more slowly.

The Denial Machine Architecture

Insurance companies employ more people to deny care than provide it. The structure is deliberate:

Layer 1: Automatic Denial
Algorithms reject claims before human eyes see them. Key triggers:

- "Experimental" or "investigational" flags

- Out-of-network providers
- "Not medically necessary" coding
- Exceeded visit limits
- Wrong diagnostic codes

My automatic denials: 67% of all claims initially rejected

Layer 2: Prior Authorization Purgatory
Even approved treatments need pre-approval. Requirements:

- Forms no one explains
- Documentation that vanishes
- Peer reviews by non-peers
- Arbitrary waiting periods
- Frequent re-authorizations

Time spent on prior authorizations: 23 hours monthly

Layer 3: Appeal Exhaustion
Each denial can be appealed, but they count on you giving up:

- First appeal: 30% success rate
- Second appeal: 45% success rate
- External review: 60% success rate
- Most people quit after first denial

My appeal record: 34 appeals filed, 23 eventually won

Layer 4: Network Narrowing
"In-network" shrinks constantly:

- Specialists leave networks
- Hospitals drop contracts
- Labs change affiliations
- Pharmacies switch preferences
- No notification until you're billed

Surprise out-of-network bills: $12,000 over three years

The Prior Authorization Torture Chamber

Prior authorization is insurance practicing medicine without a license, inserting themselves between doctor and patient, pretending cost management is care management.

The typical prior auth journey:

Week 1: Doctor prescribes medication
Week 2: Pharmacy says needs prior authorization
Week 3: Doctor's office submits paperwork
Week 4: Insurance requests additional information
Week 5: Doctor provides information
Week 6: Insurance denies as "not medically necessary"
Week 7: Doctor appeals with peer-to-peer review
Week 8: Insurance doctor (who's never seen you)

overrules your doctor
Week 9: External appeal filed
Week 10: Maybe approved, maybe not

Ten weeks suffering while bureaucracy decides if you deserve treatment your doctor already determined you need.

The Peer-to-Peer Review Scam

"Peer-to-peer" implies equals discussing. Reality: Your specialist arguing with insurance's general practitioner about specialized treatment they don't understand.

Actual peer-to-peer transcript from my records:

My neurologist: "Patient has documented POTS requiring midodrine."
Insurance doctor: "Have they tried lifestyle modifications?"
My neurologist: "Yes, extensively. Patient needs medication."
Insurance doctor: "What about compression stockings?"
My neurologist: "Already using. Insufficient alone."
Insurance doctor: "Denied. Lifestyle modifications first."

A dermatologist denying a neurologist's treatment plan. That's "peer" review.

The Formula for Denial

Insurance companies have playbooks:

The "Not Medically Necessary" Gambit
Everything is "not medically necessary" until you're dying. Preventive care that would avoid crisis? Not necessary. Early intervention? Not necessary. Maintenance treatment? Not necessary.

The "Experimental Treatment" Excuse
Treatments used for decades labeled "experimental" if expensive. Off-label use (80% of prescriptions) suddenly becomes "investigational."

The "Failed Conservative Treatment" Requirement
Must fail cheaper options first, regardless of inappropriateness. Allergic to medication? Try it anyway. Previous adverse reaction? Document it again.

The "Frequency Limitation" Trap
Physical therapy: 20 visits annually (need 52)
Mental health: 30 sessions (need weekly)
Specialist visits: 4 per year (need monthly)

When limits hit, you pay or go without.

The Appeal Letter Arsenal

After 34 appeals, I developed templates that work:

Opening Power Paragraph:
"This letter serves as formal appeal for denial of [specific treatment] dated [date], claim #[number]. This denial endangers my patient's health and contradicts established medical standards."

Evidence Bombardment Section:

- Peer-reviewed studies (with highlights)
- Medical society guidelines
- FDA approvals/indications
- Similar case precedents
- Cost comparisons (treatment vs. emergency care)

Personal Impact Statement:
"Without this treatment, I cannot [specific functions]. This has resulted in [job loss/disability/specific impacts]. Denial of medically necessary treatment constitutes bad faith insurance practice."

Closing Threat (Politely Worded):
"I expect prompt reversal of this inappropriate denial. If necessary, I will pursue external review, state insurance commission complaint, and legal remedies."

Success rate with this format: 68%

The Documentation Defense Strategy

Insurance companies count on poor record-keeping. Don't give them that advantage:

The Master Spreadsheet:

- Date of service
- Provider name
- Service provided
- Amount billed
- Amount approved
- Amount paid
- Denial reason
- Appeal status
- Notes

The Communication Log:

- Date/time of every call
- Representative name and ID
- What was promised
- Reference numbers
- Follow-up required

The Paper Trail:

- Email everything possible
- Certified mail for appeals
- Screenshot online submissions
- Record phone calls (where legal)
- Keep everything forever

This documentation saved me $18,000 in wrongly denied claims.

The Insurance Exploitation Exposé

Balance Billing Bullying:
Out-of-network provider sends massive bill. You panic, pay. Later learn about balance billing protections. Too late for refund.

The Network Bait-and-Switch:
Hospital is in-network. Surgeon is in-network. Anesthesiologist? Out-of-network. $5,000 surprise bill.

The Preventive Care Pretense:
Annual physical covered 100%. Doctor addresses existing condition during physical. Entire visit becomes diagnostic, not preventive. You owe hundreds.

The Formulary Shuffle:
Medication covered this month, not next. No notification. You discover at pharmacy when copay jumps from 30to30to300.

The Prior Authorization Reset:
Treatment approved for six months. Month seven requires new prior auth. Gap in treatment while reauthorizing already-approved treatment.

The Human Cost Calculations

Insurance companies understand actuarial science: Delay and denial save money because some people die waiting.

The death math:

- 45,000 Americans die annually from lack of insurance
- 35% of GoFundMe campaigns are for medical bills
- 66% of bankruptcies involve medical debt
- 25% of Americans skip medication due to cost
- 40% delay care due to cost

Every denial is calculated: Will this person fight or fold? Will they pay out-of-pocket or go without? Will they survive long enough to cost us more?

The Insurance Reform Revolution Required

Single-Payer Solution:
Medicare for All would eliminate:

- Prior authorizations for most care
- Network restrictions
- Surprise billing
- Medical bankruptcies
- Job lock for insurance

Public Option Alternative:
Government insurance option would:

- Create competition
- Set price benchmarks
- Ensure basic coverage
- Reduce administrative waste

Regulatory Requirements:

- Automatic approval if no response in 48 hours
- Financial penalties for inappropriate denials
- Patient representatives on review boards
- Transparent denial criteria
- Expedited appeal processes

The Guerrilla Tactics Guide

The Executive Email Carpet Bomb:
Email CEO and entire C-suite directly. Executive assistants often resolve to avoid boss involvement.

The Social Media Shame Campaign:
Twitter/Facebook posts tagging company. Public pressure works. Include claim number, keep it factual.

The Regulatory Complaint Cascade:

- State insurance commission
- Attorney general's office

- Department of Labor (for employer plans)
- Centers for Medicare/Medicaid Services

Complaints create paper trails companies hate.

The Legal Letter Leverage:
Attorney letterhead changes dynamics. Many lawyers write single letters for small fees. Often triggers immediate review.

The Media Mention Threat:
"I'm documenting this for a story about insurance denials" opens doors. Local news loves these stories.

The Alternative Funding Strategies

Pharmacy Assistance Programs:
Drug manufacturers offer free/reduced medications. Income limits higher than expected. Saved me $30,000.

Disease-Specific Foundations:
Many conditions have foundations providing financial assistance. Covered my $8,000 deductible twice.

Clinical Trials:
Free treatment plus stipends. Better care than standard sometimes.

Medical Tourism:
Hip replacement in US: $40,000 Same surgery in Spain: $7,000 including travel
Quality often comparable or better.

Crowdfunding:
Humiliating but effective. Raised $15,000 for uncovered treatments.

The Insurance Survivor Stories

Patricia's Persistence:
Denied cancer treatment as "experimental." Filed 11 appeals, contacted media, organized patient protest at insurance headquarters. Treatment approved. Now in remission. Total fight time: 7 months while having cancer.

Marcus's Malicious Compliance:
Insurance required "step therapy" - trying cheaper drugs first. Marcus tried each for exactly minimum required time, documented every side effect meticulously. Built undeniable case for needed medication. Won after 6 months.

Dr. Kim's Rebellion:
Physician spent 20 hours weekly on prior auths. Started billing insurance companies for time at lawyer rates. Sent invoices. They laughed. She organized 50 doctors to do same. Media coverage forced negotiation. Prior auths reduced 60%.

Your Insurance Battle Plan

Preparation Phase:

1. Know your policy completely
2. Understand appeal rights
3. Build documentation system
4. Research assistance programs
5. Connect with patient advocates
6. Identify regulatory agencies
7. Prepare for long war

Engagement Rules:

1. Never accept first denial
2. Document everything always
3. Escalate strategically
4. Use multiple pressure points
5. Share intelligence with others
6. Maintain emotional boundaries
7. Celebrate small victories

Escalation Ladder:

1. Internal appeal
2. External review
3. Regulatory complaints
4. Legal consultation
5. Media involvement
6. Political pressure
7. Class action participation

The Insurance Manifesto

We demand insurance that:

1. **Covers what doctors prescribe** — Medical decisions by medical professionals
2. **Approves before denying** — Assumption of coverage, not denial
3. **Processes claims promptly** — 30-day maximum resolution
4. **Eliminates prior authorization** — For established treatments
5. **Provides transparent pricing** — Know costs before treatment
6. **Removes network restrictions** — Any provider, anywhere
7. **Ends surprise billing** — One facility, one bill
8. **Covers preventive care completely** — Including chronic disease management
9. **Includes mental health equally** — No separate limits or requirements
10. **Puts patients over profits** — Healthcare, not wealth care

The Revolution Rising

Every appeal filed, every denial fought, every story shared weakens the denial machine. We're not just fighting for individual coverage — we're exposing systemic cruelty that profits from suffering.

My insurance battles cost:

- 500+ hours of my life
- $56,000 out-of-pocket with "good" insurance
- Countless treatments delayed or denied
- Immeasurable stress and trauma
- Health deterioration during delays

But also gained:

- Knowledge that helps others
- Templates that win appeals
- Networks of fighters
- Skills in healthcare navigation
- Proof that persistence pays

Your insurance battle is valid whether you win or lose. Your fight matters because it exposes the cruelty. Your story adds to the mountain of evidence that this system is unsustainable.

The revolution happens when we stop accepting denial as final answer. When we recognize that insurance companies profit from our exhaustion. When we fight not just for ourselves but for everyone denied care.

Keep fighting. Keep documenting. Keep sharing. Keep surviving.

Your care is worth more than their profit. And someday, we'll have a system that recognizes that.

That's how insurance battles become healthcare revolution.

Part II: The Hidden Healthcare System

Chapter 8: Support Groups — Where Patients Become Healers

"In hospital waiting rooms, we're strangers avoiding eye contact. In support groups, we're family who've never met, understanding each other's pain with a glance."

The Underground University of Illness

At 2 AM, when doctors are sleeping and symptoms are screaming, there's a parallel healthcare system operating. No medical degrees required, no insurance accepted, no appointments needed. Welcome to the support group universe — where patients become professors, suffering becomes curriculum, and healing happens through shared recognition that you're not alone, not crazy, and not beyond hope.

My first support group was accidental. Hospital waiting room, hour three, woman next to me noticed my compression socks and pulse oximeter. "POTS?" she asked. One word. Three letters. Instant connection.

She taught me more in 20 minutes than doctors had in two years:

- Salt loading strategies that actually work
- The brand of compression garments that don't roll
- Which ER to go to (they know POTS)
- The electrolyte drink that doesn't trigger nausea
- How to shower without fainting
- The doctor who actually listens

No copay. No prior authorization. No gaslighting. Just pure, distilled wisdom from someone who'd walked this path and survived.

The Digital Revolution of Collective Healing

Facebook groups, Reddit communities, Discord servers, WhatsApp chains — the internet transformed isolated suffering into connected healing. Geographic boundaries dissolved. Rare became common when you could find your people globally.

The numbers tell the story:

- 73% of patients use online support groups
- 91% report finding helpful information unavailable from doctors
- 67% say peer support improved their outcomes
- 45% found correct diagnosis through patient communities
- 89% feel less alone after joining groups

My digital lifelines:

- Facebook: "POTS Support Group" (47,000 members)
- Reddit: r/dysautonomia (35,000 members)
- Discord: "Spoonies Unite" (24/7 real-time support)
- Instagram: #POTSie community (visual symptom validation)
- Twitter: #NEISvoid (advocacy and awareness)

Each platform serves different needs. Facebook for detailed discussions. Reddit for anonymous questions. Discord for crisis support. Instagram for inspiration. Twitter for revolution.

The Hierarchy of Helpful Humans

Not all support groups are created equal. Through seven years of searching, I learned to recognize the types:

The Toxic Positivity Pushers:
"Good vibes only!" "Everything happens for a reason!" "You're only given what you can handle!" Run. These groups deny reality, shame struggle, and gaslight harder than bad doctors.

The Misery Competitions:
Where suffering becomes sport. "You think that's bad? Well I..." Trauma Olympics where everyone loses.

The Miracle Cure Merchants:
Every post pushing products. Essential oils, supplements, programs. MLM schemes preying on desperate people.

The Medical Echo Chambers:
Obsessing over symptoms without solutions. Anxiety amplification stations. Helpful for validation, harmful for healing.

The Balanced Biosystems:
Share struggles AND solutions. Allow venting WITH boundaries. Provide support WITHOUT enabling. Information WITH verification. These are gold.

The Unspoken Rules of Support Group Society

Every community has codes. Break them at your peril:

Rule 1: No Unsolicited Advice
"Have you tried yoga?" will get you exiled. Share what worked for you, don't prescribe for others.

Rule 2: Respect the Spectrum
From newly diagnosed to decades deep, all experiences valid. No comparing, no competing, no gatekeeping.

Rule 3: Citations Save Lives
"I read somewhere" helps no one. Link sources, name doctors, specify products. Details matter when desperate.

Rule 4: Trigger Warnings Are Courtesy
Medical trauma, treatment failures, death discussions — label heavy content. Let people choose their exposure.

Rule 5: What's Shared Stays Sacred
Screenshots without permission are betrayal. These spaces require trust. Violate it and lose community.

The Support Group Survival Guide

Finding Your Tribe:

Search strategically:

- "[Condition] + support group + [platform]"
- Check disease organization websites
- Ask doctors for recommendations (good ones know groups)
- Search hashtags on social platforms
- Check Reddit for condition-specific subs

Vet carefully:

- Read posts for two weeks before engaging
- Check group rules and moderation
- Notice tone and helpfulness
- Look for diverse experiences
- Avoid groups centered on single person

Engaging Effectively:

Start slowly:

- Introduce yourself briefly
- Read more than you post initially
- Search before asking (question probably answered)
- Thank people who help
- Share wins and struggles equally

Contribute meaningfully:

- Document what works with specifics
- Share resources generously
- Celebrate others' victories
- Offer support without fixing
- Admit what you don't know

Maintaining Boundaries:

Protect yourself:

- Limit time in groups (set timers)
- Take breaks when needed
- Don't internalize everyone's suffering
- Remember online isn't everything
- Keep some experiences private

Stay skeptical:

- Verify medical information
- Research recommended providers
- Be cautious with personal details
- Question miracle cures
- Trust but verify

The Peer Support Power Dynamics

Support groups develop hierarchies. Understanding them helps navigation:

The Elders:
Diagnosed decades ago, they've seen everything. Their experience is invaluable but sometimes outdated. Respect their journey, verify their information.

The Researchers:
Constantly sharing studies, trials, breakthroughs. Essential for cutting-edge information but can overwhelm with data. Great for specific questions.

The Cheerleaders:
Relentlessly encouraging, first to celebrate wins. Needed for morale but sometimes toxic positivity. Appreciate their energy, maintain realistic expectations.

The Crisis Counselors:
Always available for meltdowns, skilled at talking people through dark moments. Heroes but often burnt out. Support them too.

The Newcomers:
Recently diagnosed, full of questions and fear. Were you last year. Helping them helps you remember how far you've come.

The Information Marketplace

Support groups are information economies where knowledge is currency:

High-Value Information:

- Specific doctor recommendations with location
- Detailed treatment protocols with dosing
- Insurance appeal letters that worked
- Product links with discount codes
- Clinical trial opportunities
- Disability application tips

The Verification Protocol:
Never trust, always verify:

- Cross-reference medical claims
- Check doctor reviews independently
- Research products before purchasing
- Confirm insurance strategies with policy
- Validate clinical trials on official sites

I learned about Low Dose Naltrexone from support group. Researched for weeks, brought studies to doctor, tried it, life-changing. Group wisdom led to medical solution.

The Shadow Support System

Beyond formal groups exists shadow support — informal networks that save lives:

The Waiting Room Whisper Network:
Hushed conversations while waiting. "Who are you

seeing?" "Are they good?" "Try Dr. Chen instead." Information passed like contraband.

The Pharmacy Line Learning:
Comparing medications, sharing copay cards, warning about side effects. Education between "Next!" calls.

The Infusion Room Intelligence:
Hours attached to IVs create bonds. Treatment tips, doctor recommendations, insurance hacks shared between drips.

The Hospital Hallway Helpers:
Patients helping patients navigate byzantine buildings, sharing phone chargers, smuggling real food, providing witnesses for bad treatment.

The Cultural Revolution of Collective Care

Support groups aren't just information exchanges — they're cultural revolutions:

Language Liberation:
We create vocabulary for experiences medicine hasn't named. "Spoonie" for energy-limited people. "Zebra" for rare disease patients. "Painsomnia" for pain-induced insomnia. Language that validates lived experience.

Ritual Recognition:
Diagnosis anniversaries, treatment milestones, surgery send-offs. Creating ceremonies medicine ignores. Meaning-making in medical chaos.

Identity Integration:
From "patient" to "person with condition." From isolated to connected. From powerless to empowered. Groups help integrate illness without being consumed.

Advocacy Activation:
Individual suffering becomes collective action. Groups organize awareness campaigns, lobby for research, demand better care. My voice joins thousands.

The Dark Side of Desperate Connection

Not all support is supportive:

The Munchausen Manipulators:
People faking illness for attention infiltrate groups. They steal resources, emotional energy, and trust. Groups regularly unmask imposters.

The Catastrophizing Cascades:
One person's crisis triggering group-wide panic. Anxiety contagion spreading faster than virus. Moderation matters.

The Pseudoscience Proliferation:
Desperate people share desperate measures. Dangerous "treatments," conspiracy theories, anti-medicine extremism. Critical thinking crucial.

The Emotional Vampires:
Taking constantly without giving. Drama manufacturing. Energy draining. Boundaries essential for survival.

The Support Group Success Stories

Maria's Miracle Connection:
Posted symptoms in frustration. Member recognized rare genetic condition. Suggested specific test. Diagnosis confirmed after 12 years searching. Now treated, working, living.

The Insulin Rebellion:
Diabetes group discovered insurance companies denying insulin. Organized campaign, media pressure, policy changed. Thousands got life-saving medication.

David's Doctor Network:
Started spreadsheet of good doctors by location. Crowdsourced reviews. Now 5,000 entries, helping patients worldwide find care.

The Symptom Tracker Collective:
Group created app tracking symptoms across thousands. Data revealed patterns doctors missed. Research study launched based on findings.

The Professional Integration Opportunity

Forward-thinking providers recognize support group value:

Dr. Anderson's Approach:
Recommends specific groups to patients. Monitors discussions for treatment trends. Learns patient language. Says groups taught her more about living with illness than medical school.

Cleveland Clinic's Innovation:
Hosts in-person support groups. Provides meeting spaces. Doctors attend as listeners. Integrated peer support into treatment plans. Outcomes improved 34%.

The Swedish Model:
Peer support specialists employed by hospitals. Trained patients supporting current patients. Formal recognition of lived expertise. Reduced readmissions 42%.

Building Your Support Ecosystem

Layer 1: Condition-Specific Groups
Deep dive into your exact diagnosis. Maximum relevance, specific solutions.

Layer 2: Symptom Communities
Broader groups for shared symptoms. Chronic pain, fatigue, etc. Cross-pollination of strategies.

Layer 3: Local Networks
Geographic groups for provider recommendations, in-person meetups, local resources.

Layer 4: Special Interest Intersections
Groups combining condition with identity/interest. "POTS Parents," "Queer Spoonies," "Athletes with Autoimmune."

Layer 5: Crisis Support
24/7 groups for dark moments. Discord servers, WhatsApp groups with global coverage.

The Support Group Manifesto

We declare that support groups are:

1. **Essential healthcare infrastructure** — Not optional, not extra, necessary

2. **Valid sources of expertise** — Lived experience is evidence
3. **Deserving of resources** — Funding, spaces, recognition
4. **Requiring protection** — From predators, misinformation, exploitation
5. **Needing integration** — With formal healthcare, not separation
6. **Celebrating diversity** — All bodies, experiences, expressions welcome
7. **Maintaining boundaries** — Support without sacrificing self
8. **Sharing power** — Rotating leadership, democratic decisions
9. **Creating culture** — Rituals, language, meaning beyond medicine
10. **Revolutionary by existence** — Challenging medical hierarchy daily

The Truth About Support Groups

They're not consolation prizes for medical failure. They're parallel healthcare systems operating on different principles: Abundance instead of scarcity. Sharing instead of hoarding. Experience instead of theory. Connection instead of isolation.

In support groups, I found:

- Diagnosis that eluded doctors

- Treatments that transformed life
- Friends who understood without explanation
- Purpose in helping others
- Identity beyond illness
- Hope when medicine offered none

Support groups saved my life. Not metaphorically — literally. When suicide seemed logical, strangers online reminded me that tomorrow might be better. When treatment failed, they suggested alternatives. When doctors gave up, they didn't.

Your support group journey is medicine. Your contributions help others heal. Your presence matters more than you know.

The revolution happens when we recognize that patients supporting patients isn't supplementary — it's fundamental. When we understand that healing happens in community, not isolation. When we stop seeing support groups as last resort and start seeing them as first resource.

Find your people. Share your story. Learn from theirs. Heal together.

That's how support groups become healthcare transformation.

Chapter 9: Caregivers — The Invisible Army Holding Healthcare Together

"Behind every chronic illness warrior stands an exhausted caregiver whose battle scars are invisible, whose service is unpaid, and whose breaking point is treated as acceptable collateral damage."

The Shadow Workforce Nobody Counts

53 million Americans are unpaid caregivers. That's one in five adults providing $470 billion in uncompensated labor annually. We're the ghost staff of a healthcare system that would collapse in 48 hours without us, yet we remain invisible in medical charts, insurance calculations, and societal recognition.

I was a patient for seven years before my husband Mark became visible to any healthcare provider. Despite being at every appointment, managing medications, driving to ERs at 3 AM, catching me when I fainted, and losing his own health to the stress of keeping me alive, he was furniture to the medical system. Background noise. Irrelevant.

Until the day Dr. Williams asked him, "How are YOU doing?"

Mark burst into tears. Three years of accumulated exhaustion, fear, and isolation erupted in that exam room. The doctor handed him tissues and said, "You matter too."

Revolutionary words in a system that treats caregivers as unlimited resources rather than human beings with breaking points.

The Anatomy of Invisible Labor

Caregiving isn't one job — it's dozens, performed simultaneously by people never trained for any of them:

Medical Manager:

- Scheduling appointments (average 7 monthly)
- Managing medications (average 11 prescriptions)
- Tracking symptoms (daily documentation)
- Coordinating between specialists (who don't talk)

- Fighting insurance battles (20+ hours monthly)
- Researching treatments (endless)

Personal Care Assistant:

- Bathing assistance (dignity balance)
- Feeding support (when hands fail)
- Mobility help (human crutch)
- Bathroom assistance (intimate vulnerability)
- Dressing aid (preserving independence illusion)

Emotional Support Specialist:

- Crisis counselor (3 AM panic attacks)
- Motivation coach (when giving up seems logical)
- Grief companion (mourning lost life together)
- Hope holder (when patient can't)
- Normalcy creator (impossible task)

Household CEO:

- Cleaning (while exhausted)
- Cooking (special diets)
- Shopping (alone now)
- Finances (with reduced income)
- Maintenance (everything breaks when stressed)

Professional Sacrificer:

- Career derailment (60% reduce work hours)
- Promotion declination (can't travel)
- Job loss (34% leave workforce)
- Retirement depletion (average $324,000 lost)

Mark went from senior engineer to part-time contractor. $80,000 salary reduction. Career trajectory destroyed. Never complained once. The system counts this as zero economic impact.

The Stages of Caregiver Collapse

Stage 1: The Hero Phase (Months 1-6)
"I've got this." Adrenaline-fueled determination. Research obsession. Optimism that this is temporary. Sleep? Optional. Self-care? Selfish. Boundaries? Unnecessary.

Mark color-coded medication schedules, created symptom spreadsheets, built grab bars throughout our house. He was going to fix this through sheer organizational will.

Stage 2: The Reality Reckoning (Months 6-12)
Chronic means forever. Energy isn't infinite. The cavalry isn't coming. Resentment creeps in, followed by guilt about resentment. Isolation intensifies.

Mark stopped seeing friends. "How's Roi?" was the only question anyone asked. His identity evaporated. He became "Roi's husband" even to himself.

Stage 3: The Depletion Descent (Years 1-3)
Physical symptoms emerge. Emotional reserves emptied. Cognitive function impaired. Relationship strain severe. Depression common. Anxiety constant.

Mark developed hypertension, stress-induced gastritis, chronic insomnia. His doctor prescribed antidepressants. Nobody addressed the cause — unsustainable caregiving demands.

Stage 4: The Burnout Breaking (Years 3-5)
Complete exhaustion. Emotional numbness. Physical breakdown. Relationship crisis. Sometimes divorce. Sometimes abandonment. Sometimes suicide.

We almost didn't make it. The night Mark said "I can't do this anymore," I realized the system was killing both of us. Something had to change.

Stage 5: The Sustainable Rebuild (Years 5+)
Boundaries established. Help accepted. Systems created. Identity reclaimed. Relationship redefined. Not normal, but survivable.

We hired help we couldn't afford. Set caregiving hours. Created respite routines. Rebuilt relationship as partners, not patient-caregiver. Still hard. Now possible.

The Economics of Exploitation

Caregivers provide $470 billion in unpaid labor annually. If we went on strike, the healthcare system would collapse before lunch. Yet:

- No compensation for time
- No Social Security credits
- No unemployment insurance
- No workers' compensation
- No retirement contributions
- No health insurance
- No sick days
- No vacation
- No overtime
- No breaks

The financial devastation:

- Average caregiver spends $7,000 annually out-of-pocket
- 48% deplete savings completely
- 23% lose homes
- 34% accumulate credit card debt
- 67% struggle with basic expenses
- 45% cut own medical care

Mark calculated his economic loss: 560,000inreducedearnings,560,000inreducedearnin gs,180,000 in lost retirement contributions, 45,000inout-of-pocketcosts.Total:45,000inout-of-pocketcosts.Total:785,000. Recognition from system: Zero.

The Health Theft Nobody Measures

Caregiving literally kills:

- 63% higher mortality rate than non-caregivers
- 23% higher risk of stroke
- 40% higher risk of depression
- 51% higher risk of anxiety
- Immune function decreased 15%
- Cellular aging accelerated 9 years

Mark aged a decade in three years. Gray hair, weight gain, chronic pain from lifting me, hypertension from stress, depression from isolation. His health sacrificed for mine. The system considers this acceptable.

The Relationship Demolition

Chronic illness doesn't just affect individuals — it detonates relationships:

Marriage Mortality:

- 75% divorce rate for chronic illness
- Higher if wife is sick (men leave more)
- Increases with disability severity
- Peaks at year three

We survived, barely. Couples therapy saved us. Learning to be partners, not caregiver-patient. Scheduling intimacy like medication. Finding each other again in the wreckage.

Family Fractures:

- Siblings resentful of attention imbalance
- Parents exhausted by adult children's needs
- Children parentified before ready
- Extended family disappears

My sister stopped calling. "It's always about your illness." She wasn't wrong. Crisis consumed everything. Relationships require energy we didn't have.

Friendship Fadeout:

- 68% of caregivers lose friendships
- Social invitations stop
- "How is [patient]?" only question
- Own struggles minimized
- Isolation becomes default

Mark's friends evaporated. Couldn't commit to plans. Conversations became medical updates. His problems seemed trivial compared to illness. Loneliness compounded exhaustion.

The Gender Expectations Trap

Women provide 66% of caregiving but receive less support:

- Expected to sacrifice without complaint
- Judged for seeking help
- Paid less when working
- Career impact greater
- Health consequences worse

When men are caregivers, they're heroes. When women are caregivers, they're doing their duty. Mark got praised for basic tasks. Female caregivers get criticized for not doing more.

Cultural expectations multiply burden:

- Latina women expected to provide all care personally
- Asian families shame outside help
- Black women carry "strong" stereotype preventing help-seeking
- Rural communities lack any support services
- Religious communities offer prayers, not practical help

The Children Nobody Sees

1.4 million children are caregivers. Kids managing parents' medications, translating at appointments, missing school for emergencies, growing up too fast.

Their invisible sacrifices:

- Academic performance drops 30%
- College attendance decreases 40%
- Mental health issues triple
- Social development impaired
- Career choices limited
- Childhood stolen

These children become adults who don't know how to not caretake. Hypervigilance becomes personality. Anxiety their baseline. The system pretends they don't exist.

The Professional Caregiver Paradox

Paid caregivers — CNAs, home health aides, personal care assistants — provide essential services for poverty wages:

- Average wage: $12/hour
- No benefits typical
- High injury rates

- Emotional labor uncompensated
- Turnover 82% annually

We finally hired help. Maria, our aide, was incredible. She made $11/hour to do work that saved my life and Mark's sanity. The agency charged $35/hour. She couldn't afford health insurance while providing healthcare.

The Support That Doesn't Exist

Respite care: Waitlists years long, costs prohibitive, quality questionable
Support groups: Rare, inaccessible, scheduled when caregiving
Financial assistance: Minimal, complex applications, humiliating requirements
Mental health services: Expensive, not covered, no time to attend
Training: Assumes medical knowledge, ignores emotional aspects
Recognition: Absolutely none

The system's message: Figure it out yourself.

The International Inspiration

Other countries recognize caregivers:

Germany: Caregivers receive pension credits, paid leave, training, respite care
Japan: Long-term care insurance covers family caregivers
Australia: Carer Payment provides income support
UK: Carer's Allowance, though inadequate, acknowledges role
Nordic countries: Comprehensive support including salary, training, respite

America: Thoughts and prayers. Bootstrap pulling. Individual responsibility for collective crisis.

The Caregiver Revolution Rising

Change is happening, slowly:

The RAISE Act: Recognizing caregivers in healthcare planning (unfunded mandate)
Employer Support: Some companies offering caregiver leave (rare)
Technology Solutions: Apps connecting caregivers, sharing resources
Advocacy Organizations: Fighting for recognition, resources, rights
Caregiver Resource Centers: Providing information, support, referrals

But revolution requires more than incremental change.

The Sustainable Caregiving Model

We developed survival strategies:

Scheduled Boundaries:

- Caregiving hours: 8 AM - 8 PM
- Emergency exceptions only
- Night duty rotates
- Weekends partially protected
- Vacation mandatory

Distributed Labor:

- Hired help (sacrificed everything else)
- Friends assigned specific tasks
- Online grocery delivery
- Medication mail-order
- Virtual appointments when possible

Identity Preservation:

- Mark maintains one hobby
- Separate therapy sessions
- Individual friend time
- Career continuity somehow
- Relationship time scheduled

Communication Protocols:

- Daily check-ins about needs
- Weekly relationship meeting
- Monthly capacity assessment
- Permission to say "I can't"
- Celebration of small wins

Respite Requirements:

- Two hours daily minimum
- One day weekly off
- One weekend monthly away
- One week annually vacation
- Guilt-free enforcement

The Technology Bridge

Apps and devices reducing burden:

Medication Management:

- Automated dispensers
- Reminder apps
- Interaction checkers
- Refill coordination

Communication Tools:

- Care coordination apps
- Video visit platforms
- Symptom trackers

- Emergency alert systems

Support Networks:

- Caregiver communities online
- Resource sharing platforms
- Respite exchange programs
- Virtual support groups

Administrative Assistance:

- Insurance navigation tools
- Document management
- Appointment scheduling
- Bill paying services

Technology doesn't replace human care but enables sustainability.

The Caregiver's Caregiver

Who cares for the caregiver? Usually nobody. But should be everybody:

Healthcare Providers:

- Ask about caregiver wellbeing
- Provide resources proactively
- Recognize signs of burnout
- Include in care planning
- Validate their expertise

Family/Friends:

- Offer specific help
- Don't wait to be asked
- Show up consistently
- Ask about THEM
- Provide respite

Employers:

- Flexible scheduling
- Caregiver leave
- EAP resources
- Understanding culture
- Remote options

Society:

- Recognition of value
- Financial support
- Respite infrastructure
- Training programs
- Policy prioritization

The Caregiver Bill of Rights

We declare that caregivers have the right to:

1. **Recognition as essential healthcare providers**
2. **Compensation for labor provided**
3. **Training for tasks expected**
4. **Respite without guilt**
5. **Physical and mental health support**

6. Boundaries without judgment
7. Identity beyond caregiving
8. Resources for sustainability
9. Community and connection
10. Life worth living too

The Letter to My Caregiver

Mark,

You saved my life. Not once but daily. For seven years, you've been my anchor in the storm, my translator in medical chaos, my hope when I had none.

You've sacrificed career, health, friendships, dreams. You've cleaned up things that shouldn't need cleaning, held me through seizures of frustration, fought battles I was too weak to fight.

The system doesn't see you. Insurance doesn't count you. Society doesn't value you.

But I do. We do. Every patient knows that without you, we don't survive.

You're not just my caregiver. You're my hero. And heroes deserve more than exhaustion as reward.

The Truth About Caregiving

It's love in action. It's sacrifice beyond reason. It's strength that shouldn't be required. It's invisible labor that holds everything together.

Caregivers aren't saints or martyrs. They're humans pushed beyond human limits by systems that extract their labor while denying their humanity.

The healthcare system is built on the backs of unpaid caregivers. Our exhaustion subsidizes inadequate services. Our breakdown is acceptable collateral damage.

But we're rising. Organizing. Demanding recognition, resources, revolution.

Every caregiver who sets boundaries models sustainability. Every employer who provides support changes culture. Every policy that recognizes caregivers transforms systems.

The revolution happens when we stop accepting caregiver burnout as inevitable. When we recognize that caring for caregivers is caring for patients. When we understand that sustainable caregiving requires societal support.

To every caregiver reading this: You matter. Your needs are valid. Your limits are real. Your contribution is heroic. Your breakdown is not required.

To everyone else: See the caregivers. Support them. Recognize them. Value them. Fight for them.

Because when caregivers fall, we all fall.

That's how supporting caregivers becomes healthcare revolution.

Chapter 10: Alternative Medicine — When Desperation Meets Hope at the Intersection of Science and Faith

"The alternative medicine industry thrives not because people are gullible, but because conventional medicine leaves them so desperate they'll try anything, pay anything, believe anything that offers hope."

The $82 Billion Cry for Help

Alternative medicine generates $82 billion annually in America. That's not ignorance spending — it's desperation investing. Every dollar represents someone failed by conventional medicine, seeking healing wherever it might hide.

I contributed approximately $30,000 to that number over seven years. Acupuncture, naturopathy, functional medicine, energy healing, supplements, devices, programs, protocols. Some helped, most didn't, all took money I didn't have from hope I couldn't afford to lose.

But here's what critics miss: When you're drowning, you grab any rope thrown, even if it might be a snake. When medicine offers nothing, something — even if it's placebo — becomes everything.

The Hierarchy of Alternative Attempts

Tier 1: The Almost-Mainstream
Acupuncture, chiropractic, massage therapy. Insurance sometimes covers. Some evidence base. Medical doctors occasionally recommend.

My acupuncture experience: 100/session,twiceweeklyforthreemonths.Helpedwith pain,improvedenergyslightly.Notcurebutgenuinereli ef.Worththe100/session,twiceweeklyforthreemonths .Helpedwithpain,improvedenergyslightly.Notcurebut genuinerelief.worththe2,400? When nothing else worked, yes.

Tier 2: The Supplement Supermarket
Vitamins, minerals, herbs, enzymes, probiotics. The average chronic illness patient takes 12+ supplements. Monthly cost: $200-500.

My supplement graveyard: Turmeric, CoQ10, magnesium, B-complex, D3, omega-3, probiotics, digestive enzymes, adaptogenic herbs, amino acids, methylation support, mitochondrial cocktails. Some helped (magnesium for muscle cramps), most expensive urine.

Tier 3: The Functional Frontier
Functional medicine, integrative medicine, naturopathy. Comprehensive testing, systems approach, root cause investigation. Not covered by insurance. Initial consultation: $500-1,500.

My functional medicine journey: $3,000 in testing revealed gut dysbiosis, methylation issues, mitochondrial dysfunction. Treatment protocol helped 30%. Expensive but more thorough than any conventional doctor.

Tier 4: The Energy Esoterica
Reiki, healing touch, quantum healing, crystal therapy, sound healing. Zero scientific basis. Powerful placebo potential.

My energy healing experiment: 150forReikisession.Feltnothingduring,sleptbetteraft er.Placebo?Probably.Butbestsleepinmonthswaswor th150forReikisession.Feltnothingduring,sleptbettera fter.Placebo?Probably.Butbestsleepinmonthswaswo rth150.

Tier 5: The Dangerous Desperate
Miracle cures, stem cell tourism, unregulated treatments, black salve, MMS (bleach), dangerous detoxes. Where hope meets harm.

Never went here, but understood the temptation. When death seems certain, even dangerous chances seem logical.

The Psychology of Alternative Appeal

Why do intelligent people try unproven treatments?

The Time Investment:
Alternative practitioners spend TIME. Initial consultations often 90 minutes. Follow-ups 45 minutes. They listen, investigate, consider whole person.

Compare: 15-minute conventional appointments where doctors interrupt after 11 seconds.

The Validation Value:
Alternative practitioners rarely say "it's all in your

head." They validate suffering, acknowledge complexity, offer hope. Even if treatments don't work, being believed heals something.

The Control Illusion:
Conventional medicine happens TO you. Alternative medicine happens WITH you. Dietary changes, lifestyle modifications, supplement protocols — you're doing something, not just waiting.

The Explanation Appetite:
"Your chakras are blocked" might be nonsense, but it's an explanation. When conventional medicine offers only "idiopathic" (we don't know), even false explanations feel better than none.

The Hope Market:
Conventional medicine often offers management, not cure. Alternative medicine promises transformation. False hope? Often. But hope nonetheless.

The Practitioner Spectrum

The True Believers:
Genuinely believe they're helping. Often helped themselves with method they're selling. Passionate, convincing, sometimes right.

My chiropractor genuinely believed adjustments would cure POTS. They didn't, but his certainty was infectious. Three months of hope worth $1,200.

The Scientific Straddlers:
Medical training plus alternative methods. Foot in both worlds. Often best option.

Dr. Chen, MD and licensed acupuncturist. Understood both languages. Provided integrated care that actually helped.

The Sophisticated Scammers:
Know it doesn't work. Don't care. Expensive offices, complex protocols, sciencey language. Prey on desperate wealthy.

The "quantum healer" who charged $500 to wave hands over me while discussing cellular vibrations. Knew immediately but so desperate I completed session.

The Dangerous Delusional:
Believe conventional medicine is conspiracy. Discourage proven treatments. Promote dangerous alternatives. Kill people with conviction.

Met one who insisted I stop all medications, use only herbs. Would have killed me. Ran away fast.

The Evidence Examination

Some alternative treatments have evidence:

Acupuncture:

- Effective for certain pain conditions
- Helps some nausea
- May improve some headaches
- Mechanisms unclear but effects real

Meditation/Mindfulness:

- Reduces stress markers
- Improves pain tolerance
- Enhances immune function
- Changes brain structure

Certain Supplements:

- Vitamin D for deficiency
- B12 for anemia
- Magnesium for deficiency
- Probiotics for specific conditions

Yoga/Tai Chi:

- Improves balance
- Reduces fall risk
- Enhances flexibility
- Decreases anxiety

But most alternatives lack evidence because research is expensive and can't be patented.

The Placebo Power Reality

Placebo effect is real medicine:

- 30% average improvement from placebo
- Brain imaging shows actual changes
- Endorphins released
- Inflammation reduced
- Immune function enhanced

If sugar pill makes you 30% better through belief, is that fake healing or real improvement? Philosophy aside, 30% improvement changes lives.

My relationship with placebo evolved. Initially insulted by suggestion symptoms were "placebo responsive." Now? If expensive water blessed by shamans improves symptoms 20%, I'll drink expensive water.

The Integration Innovation

Best outcomes combine conventional and complementary:

Cancer Centers:
Leading centers now offer acupuncture for chemo nausea, meditation for anxiety, massage for pain. Not replacing treatment but enhancing.

Pain Clinics:
Multimodal approaches including physical therapy,

psychology, acupuncture, medications. Better outcomes than single interventions.

Cleveland Clinic's Center for Integrative Medicine:
Offers acupuncture, massage, yoga, supplements alongside conventional care. Patients report higher satisfaction, better outcomes.

The Regulation Roulette

Supplements are barely regulated:

- No pre-market approval required
- No proof of efficacy needed
- No standardized dosing
- No interaction testing
- No adverse event monitoring

The Wild West where anything goes until people die.

My supplement scares:

- "Natural" thyroid supplement contained actual thyroid hormone
- Herbal blend interacted with medication
- Probiotic contaminated with harmful bacteria
- CBD oil contained no CBD
- Expensive vitamins were compressed sawdust

Now I only buy third-party tested, GMP-certified, independently verified. Costs more. Worth it.

The Cultural Context

Different cultures, different "alternatives":

Traditional Chinese Medicine:
Mainstream in China, alternative here. 3,000 years of empirical observation dismissed because not double-blind tested.

Ayurveda:
India's traditional system. Sophisticated, systematic, sometimes effective. Dismissed as woo in West.

Indigenous Medicine:
Plant medicines that became pharmaceuticals. Wisdom holders marginalized while companies profit from their knowledge.

What's "alternative" depends on who's defining mainstream.

The Insurance Inequality

Insurance covers:

- Opioids that kill (but profitable)
- Surgeries that might help (very profitable)

- Medications with severe side effects (extremely profitable)

Insurance doesn't cover:

- Acupuncture that helps (not profitable)
- Nutrition counseling that prevents (reduces profit)
- Supplements that support (can't patent)

The system pushes people toward alternatives by making proven complementary treatments inaccessible.

The Desperate Decision Tree

When conventional medicine fails:

Stage 1: Accepted Alternatives
Try acupuncture, chiropractic, massage. Tell doctor. Insurance might cover.

Stage 2: Expanded Experiments
Naturopaths, functional medicine, extensive supplements. Don't tell doctor. Pay cash.

Stage 3: Esoteric Exploration
Energy healing, homeopathy, medical mediums. Tell nobody. Credit cards.

Stage 4: Dangerous Desperation
Stem cell tourism, unregulated treatments, internet protocols. Risk everything.

I reached Stage 3.5. Almost tried stem cells in Panama. Cost: $30,000. Risk: unknown. Desperation: absolute. Stopped by friend who'd been harmed by similar treatment.

The Alternative Medicine Survival Guide

Research Rigorously:

- PubMed for studies
- Examine.com for supplement evidence
- ConsumerLab for quality testing
- QuackWatch for scam alerts

Verify Practitioners:

- Check licenses
- Verify credentials
- Read reviews critically
- Ask for references
- Trust your instincts

Test Carefully:

- One treatment at a time
- Document everything
- Set spending limits

- Define success metrics
- Have exit strategy

Integrate Intelligently:

- Tell all providers everything
- Check interactions
- Monitor closely
- Adjust as needed
- Stop if harmful

The Success Stories and Cautionary Tales

Success: Lisa's Lyme Recovery
Conventional treatment failed. Functional medicine doctor found co-infections, treated comprehensively. 80% improved. Cost: $50,000. "Bankruptcy or death — easy choice."

Success: Marcus's Migraine Management
Acupuncture plus elimination diet plus magnesium. Migraines reduced 70%. Monthly cost: $400. "Cheaper than ER visits."

Caution: Jennifer's Juice Disaster
Stopped chemo for juice cleanses. Cancer progressed. Returned to conventional treatment too late. Died believing she'd failed protocol, not that protocol failed her.

Caution: David's Detox Damage
Extreme detox protocol caused kidney damage. Hospitalized. Permanent dysfunction. Provider disappeared. No recourse.

The Provider Perspective

Dr. Sarah Anderson, integrative medicine physician:

"I went alternative because conventional medicine failed my own chronic illness. Now I bridge both worlds. Some alternatives are nonsense. Some are tomorrow's mainstream. Dismissing everything alternative is as foolish as believing everything alternative."

The Future of Integration

Medicine is slowly recognizing value:

Research Increasing:
NIH funds complementary medicine research. Studies revealing mechanisms, benefits, risks.

Education Expanding:
Medical schools teaching about supplements, acupuncture, meditation. New generation more open.

Integration Advancing:
Major medical centers adding integrative services. Insurance coverage slowly expanding.

The Alternative Medicine Manifesto

We demand:

1. **Research into all healing modalities** — Not just profitable ones
2. **Regulation ensuring safety** — Without eliminating access
3. **Insurance coverage for proven alternatives** — Acupuncture, nutrition, supplements
4. **Integration not segregation** — Complementary alongside conventional
5. **Cultural respect** — Traditional medicine wisdom valued
6. **Practitioner accountability** — Standards, oversight, recourse
7. **Honest information** — Benefits and risks transparent
8. **Patient choice** — Informed consent for all approaches
9. **Affordable access** — Healing shouldn't require wealth
10. **Hope with honesty** — Promise possibility, not miracles

The Truth About Alternative Medicine

It exists because conventional medicine fails too many. It thrives on desperation. It offers hope where none exists. It sometimes helps, sometimes harms, always costs.

But dismissing it entirely misses the point. People seeking alternatives aren't stupid — they're suffering. They're not gullible — they're desperate. They're not anti-science — they're failed by science.

My $30,000 alternative journey taught me:

- Some helps (acupuncture, magnesium, meditation)
- Most doesn't (energy healing, expensive supplements)
- All provides something conventional medicine doesn't (time, hope, agency)
- None replaces proven treatments
- Integration beats segregation

The revolution isn't choosing alternative OR conventional. It's demanding AND. Both. Together. Integrated. Because healing happens in many ways, through many modalities, and limiting options limits outcomes.

Your alternative journey is valid. Your experiments understandable. Your hope admirable. Your skepticism warranted. Your integration optimal.

The future of medicine isn't alternative versus conventional — it's the best of both, the wisdom to know which, and the access to choose.

That's how alternative medicine becomes integrated healing.

Part III: The Human Cost

Chapter 11: Mental Health in Medical Crisis — When Your Mind Bears the Weight Your Body Can't Carry

"They treat the body and ignore the mind, as if chronic illness only affects organs, not the person living with them. But mental health isn't separate from physical health — it's the foundation that keeps us alive when our bodies try to kill us."

The Epidemic Inside the Epidemic

87% of chronic illness patients experience depression. 73% have anxiety. 45% contemplate suicide. 25% attempt. These aren't character flaws or weakness — they're predictable psychological responses to sustained medical trauma.

Yet mental health remains healthcare's neglected stepchild. We'll spend millions keeping bodies alive while ignoring minds dying. Insurance covers endless physical procedures but limits therapy to 20 sessions annually. ERs stabilize cardiac crisis but discharge psychiatric crisis. We have cardiologists for hearts, neurologists for brains, but nobody for the human experiencing both.

I attempted suicide on day 1,847 of my illness. Not from pain, though pain was constant. Not from disability, though independence was gone. From the exhaustion of fighting systems that demanded I prove I deserved to live while making living impossible.

The ER pumped my stomach, lectured about "choosing life," and discharged me to the same circumstances that made death seem logical. No therapy referral. No medication adjustment. No recognition that chronic illness had created acute crisis.

That's when I learned: The healthcare system will save your life but won't help you want to live it.

The Stages of Psychological Collapse

Stage 1: The Denial Defense (Months 1-3)
"This is temporary." Your mind protects you with optimism. Depression hasn't arrived because you haven't accepted permanence. Anxiety exists but feels proportional. Hope is genuine, not desperate.

I spent three months certain I'd wake up recovered. Planned future assuming health. Mind protecting itself from truth it couldn't yet process.

Stage 2: The Anger Uprising (Months 3-12)
Rage arrives as denial dissolves. At your body for betraying. At doctors for failing. At God for allowing. At healthy people for existing. At yourself for everything.

Anger was rocket fuel. Powered research, advocacy, survival. But rockets burn out, and anger without outlet becomes depression's preview.

Stage 3: The Bargaining Burnout (Years 1-2)
"If I just try hard enough..." Desperate deals with universe. Perfect compliance with treatment. Elimination diets. Exercise despite exhaustion. Positive thinking as medicine.

I became wellness warrior. Meditation, gratitude journals, visualization. Mind over matter. Spoiler: Matter won.

Stage 4: The Depression Descent (Years 2-4)
When bargaining fails, darkness arrives. Not sadness — emptiness. Not grief — numbness. Colors fade. Food tastes gray. Love feels distant. Death seems logical.

Depression with chronic illness isn't just chemical imbalance — it's realistic assessment of circumstances. When life is objectively terrible, feeling terrible is rational response.

Stage 5: The Acceptance Ambiguity (Years 4+)
Not accepting illness — accepting that fighting it alone won't work. That mental health needs treatment like physical health. That surviving requires more than medical intervention.

Acceptance isn't giving up. It's strategic surrender that enables sustainable resistance.

The Suicide Mathematics

Chronic illness increases suicide risk 400%. The calculation is coldly logical:

Pain (constant) + Exhaustion (profound) + Financial destruction (ongoing) + Relationship loss (accumulating) + Treatment failure (repeated) + Hope depletion (accelerating) = Death as solution

I made lists:

- Reasons to live (shrinking)
- Reasons to die (growing)
- People who'd miss me (but be relieved)
- Things I'd miss (that I couldn't do anyway)

The math kept equaling exit.

What saved me wasn't inspirational quotes or hotline calls. It was rage at systems that expected this outcome. Suicide would be their victory, my final compliance with their assessment that chronically ill lives aren't worth living.

I lived out of spite. Then slowly found better reasons.

The Medical Trauma Nobody Names

Medical PTSD is real:

- 25% of ICU survivors develop PTSD
- 30% of chronic illness patients have trauma symptoms
- Repeated medical experiences create complex trauma

- Symptoms dismissed as "anxiety about health"

My triggers:

- Hospital smell (instant panic)
- Blood pressure cuffs (arm bruises remembered)
- Waiting rooms (accumulated dread)
- White coats (dismissal uniform)
- Medical forms (bureaucratic violence)
- Phone ringing (bad news delivery)

Every medical encounter risked retraumatization. Seeking help hurt. The cure was killing.

The Anxiety Architecture

Chronic illness anxiety isn't irrational fear — it's pattern recognition:

Body Anxiety:
Every sensation potential crisis. Is this headache normal or stroke? Chest pain or heart attack? Fatigue or organ failure? Hypervigilance to bodies that betray randomly.

Medical Anxiety:
Will they believe me? Dismiss me? Harm me? Help me? Every appointment Russian roulette.

Financial Anxiety:
Will insurance cover? Can I afford copays? What if I can't work? Bankruptcy lurking.

Future Anxiety:
Will it get worse? Will treatments stop working? Will I die young? Will I die suffering?

Existential Anxiety:
Who am I if not capable? What's life's meaning in limitation? Do I matter if I can't contribute?

Anxiety wasn't disorder — it was realistic response to uncertain circumstances.

The Grief Nobody Acknowledges

Chronic illness grief is complicated:

- Grieving yourself while still alive
- Mourning futures that won't happen
- Loss without closure
- Grief retriggered by each new limitation

I grieved:

- The athlete I was
- The doctor I'd planned to be
- The spontaneous person who died
- The independence I'd never regain
- The simplicity I'd never know again

But saying "I'm grieving" prompted "At least you're alive!" As if gratitude for survival negates grief for what survival costs.

The Therapy That Doesn't Exist

Finding mental health support for medical trauma:

Problem 1: Therapists who don't understand
"Have you tried thinking positively?"
"Maybe accepting limitations would help"
"Focus on what you can do, not can't"

Toxic positivity from professionals who should know better.

Problem 2: Inaccessible care
Can't drive to appointments. No energy for weekly sessions. Insurance limits visits. Copays unaffordable.

Problem 3: Medical model mismatch
CBT assumes thoughts create feelings. But when circumstances are objectively terrible, negative thoughts are accurate assessment, not cognitive distortion.

Problem 4: Separation of mental and physical
Psychiatrists who won't consider medical contributions. Medical doctors who won't address

psychological impacts. Nobody treating whole person.

Finally found therapist specializing in chronic illness. She understood that positive thinking wouldn't cure POTS, that grief was appropriate, that anger was justified, that suicide ideation was symptom of circumstances, not character.

The Medication Minefield

Psychiatric medications with chronic illness are complicated:

Interaction Chaos:
Antidepressants affecting heart rate (already dysregulated)
Anxiety medications causing fatigue (already exhausted)
Mood stabilizers affecting blood pressure (already unstable)

Side Effect Amplification:
Normal side effects become unbearable when added to existing symptoms. Mild nausea becomes unable to eat. Slight fatigue becomes bedbound.

The Chemical Scapegoat:
Everything blamed on psych meds. New symptom? Must be antidepressant. Ignore advancing illness.

The Stigma Spiral:
Taking psychiatric medication seen as admission symptoms are psychological. Proof you're "crazy" not sick.

Took me two years to try antidepressants. Three more to find one that helped without harming. SSRI for depression that was absolutely biological, not character flaw.

The Support Group Psychology

Mental health happens in community:

Validation Value:
Others saying "me too" heals in ways therapy can't. Not alone. Not crazy. Not weak.

Practical Strategies:
Learning how others cope. What helps. What hurts. Collective wisdom surpassing professional knowledge.

Purpose Through Helping:
Supporting others provides meaning. Your suffering helps someone. Purpose when you thought you had none.

Reality Checking:
Is this normal chronic illness experience or crisis needing intervention? Group knows difference.

Online support groups saved my life repeatedly. 3 AM panic attacks met with immediate support. Suicide ideation talked through. Hope shared when mine depleted.

The Family Mental Health Fallout

Chronic illness doesn't just break individual minds — it fractures family psychology:

Caregiver Depression:
Mark developed moderate depression year two. His therapist said 70% of caregivers need mental health treatment. None receive it automatically.

Sibling Resentment:
My sister needed therapy to process anger at attention my illness required. Valid feelings that needed space.

Parental Grief:
Parents mourn children's lost futures. Blame themselves for genetics. Age faster under stress.

Children's Anxiety:
Kids with chronically ill parents show higher anxiety, depression, behavioral problems. They need support but rarely receive.

Family therapy should be standard with chronic illness diagnosis. Never is.

The Workplace Psychology

Chronic illness creates workplace mental health crisis:

Imposter Syndrome:
Am I faking wellness to keep job? Faking illness when needing accommodation? Can't win.

Disclosure Dilemmas:
Tell employer and risk discrimination? Hide and risk performance issues? No good options.

Productivity Pressure:
Pushing through symptoms to prove worth. Making illness worse to keep income.

Identity Crisis:
When career defines you, losing capacity means losing self.

I went from rising star to liability. The psychological toll of professional death while physically alive nearly killed me.

The Technology and Mental Health

Digital tools helping:

Meditation Apps:
Calm, Headspace, Insight Timer. Accessible when leaving bed impossible.

Teletherapy:
BetterHelp, Talkspace. Therapy from bed. Game-changer for homebound.

Mood Tracking:
Daylio, eMoods. Pattern recognition. Medication monitoring.

Crisis Support:
Crisis Text Line. 24/7 help. Saved me multiple times.

Virtual Support Groups:
Facebook, Discord, Reddit. Community always available.

Technology doesn't replace in-person but enables access when illness prevents traditional care.

The Mental Health Revolution Required

Integration Innovation:

- Mental health screening at every medical appointment
- Therapists embedded in medical teams

- Psychiatrists who understand medical complexity
- Automatic mental health referrals with chronic diagnosis

Access Advancement:

- Insurance parity actually enforced
- Unlimited therapy for medical trauma
- Teletherapy universally covered
- Group therapy options expanded

Training Transformation:

- Medical schools teaching psychological impact
- Therapy programs including medical trauma
- Integrated treatment approaches
- Whole-person medicine

The Survival Strategies

What actually helped:

Radical Acceptance:
Not accepting illness as good but as reality. Energy spent fighting reality is energy stolen from living.

Micro-Dosing Hope:
Not hoping for cure but for good hour. Good day. Good moment. Small hopes achievable.

Meaning Making:
Finding purpose in illness. Helping others. Writing. Advocating. Transforming suffering into service.

Boundary Building:
Saying no to toxic positivity. Limiting exposure to healthy people's problems. Protecting emotional energy.

Professional Help:
Therapy. Medication. Support groups. Using every tool available.

Creative Expression:
Writing, art, music. Externalizing internal chaos. Creating beauty from breakdown.

The Mental Health Manifesto

We demand:

1. **Recognition that chronic illness causes mental illness** — Not weakness
2. **Automatic mental health support with medical diagnosis** — Standard care
3. **Insurance coverage for unlimited therapy** — Trauma doesn't have session limits
4. **Integration of mental and physical healthcare** — One person, one system
5. **Training for providers in medical trauma** — Specialized knowledge needed

6. **Family mental health support** — Illness affects everyone
7. **Workplace mental health accommodations** — Psychological needs matter
8. **Peer support funding** — Lived experience helps
9. **Crisis resources specifically for chronic illness** — Unique needs
10. **Hope without toxic positivity** — Realistic support

The Truth About Mental Health and Chronic Illness

Your depression is not character flaw — it's predictable response to impossible circumstances. Your anxiety is not irrational — it's pattern recognition in chaotic system. Your suicide ideation is not weakness — it's exhaustion from fighting alone.

Mental health with chronic illness isn't about positive thinking or acceptance or gratitude. It's about survival. It's about finding reasons to continue when continuing seems impossible. It's about building life worth living within limitations that feel unlivable.

My mental health journey paralleled physical: Denied, dismissed, delayed, but eventually treated.

Therapy, medication, support groups, purpose, creativity, community. Still struggle. Still survive. Still here.

Your mental health matters as much as physical. Your psychological symptoms are as real as physical ones. Your need for help is not weakness.

The revolution happens when we stop separating mind from body. When we recognize that chronic illness breaks both and both need healing. When mental healthcare becomes standard, not luxury.

Seek help. Take medication if needed. Join support groups. Express yourself. Set boundaries. Find purpose. Choose life, even when life feels impossible.

Your mind is keeping you alive when your body tries to kill you. It deserves care, support, recognition, and healing.

That's how mental health becomes medical revolution.

Chapter 12: Financial Toxicity — When Healthcare Costs More

Than Money Can Measure

"Medical bankruptcy isn't just financial failure — it's the system declaring that your life is worth less than their profit, that healing is luxury, and that poverty is acceptable side effect of illness."

The American Healthcare Lottery

In America, your zip code predicts your health more than your genetic code. Your bank account determines your treatment more than your diagnosis. Your job decides your survival more than your prognosis.

I had "good" insurance. College-educated. Middle-class. Saved responsibly. Still went bankrupt. Not dramatically, with lawyers and courtrooms, but slowly, selling everything, draining retirement, maxing credit cards, begging for help, choosing between medications and mortgage.

The numbers tell one story:

- $126,000 in medical debt over seven years
- $420,000 in lost income
- $85,000 in retirement savings liquidated

- $45,000 in credit card debt accumulated
- $30,000 borrowed from family
- $15,000 raised through GoFundMe

The reality tells another: Financial toxicity doesn't just take money — it takes dignity, security, future, hope. It transforms illness from medical crisis to economic catastrophe, adding trauma to trauma, making healing impossible when you're drowning in debt.

The Hidden Costs Nobody Calculates

Medical bills are just the visible tip of financial toxicity's iceberg:

The Transportation Trap:

- Gas to appointments: $200/month
- Parking at hospitals: $15-30/visit
- Uber when unable to drive: $50/trip
- Medical transport: Not covered
- Wear on vehicle: Accelerated

Three appointments weekly, specialists an hour away. Transportation cost more than some medications.

The Accommodation Amendments:

- Shower chair: $150

- Grab bars: $200
- Raised toilet seat: $75
- Bedroom commode: $100
- Wheelchair: $500
- Ramp installation: $2,000
- Stair lift: $5,000

Making home livable with disability: $10,000 minimum. Insurance covers nothing. Safety becomes luxury.

The Dietary Demands:

- Special diet foods: $300/month extra
- Supplements not covered: $200/month
- Meal delivery when can't cook: $400/month
- Nutrition consults not covered: $150/session

Eating for health costs more than eating for survival. Ramen is cheap. Organic anti-inflammatory diet isn't.

The Communication Costs:

- Phone bills for insurance battles: Extra $50/month
- Internet for research/telehealth: $100/month
- Printer for documentation: $200
- Paper, ink, postage: $30/month

Fighting for care requires infrastructure. Being sick is expensive administrative job.

The Clothing Casualties:

- Compression garments: $300 each, need multiple
- Easy-dress adaptive clothing: Triple regular cost
- Non-slip shoes: $150
- Multiple sizes for weight fluctuation: Complete wardrobe rebuilds

Looking "normal" costs more when your body isn't.

The Income Execution

Chronic illness is career death sentence:

The Productivity Plunge:
Can't work full-time. Reduced to part-time. Then freelance. Then nothing. Income evaporates while expenses explode.

My trajectory:

- Year 1: $75,000 salary
- Year 2: $45,000 (reduced hours)
- Year 3: $20,000 (freelance)
- Year 4-7: $0-5,000 (occasional writing)

From comfortable to catastrophic in 36 months.

The Benefits Bloodbath:
Lose job, lose insurance. COBRA costs

1,800/month. Marketplaceplanswithworsecoveragecost1,800/month. Marketplaceplanswithworsecoveragecost800/month. Sick tax for being too sick to work.

The Disability Denial:
Applied for disability. Denied. Appealed. Denied. Hired lawyer (30% of any back pay). Finally approved after three years. Monthly benefit: $1,100. Poverty wage for being disabled.

The Career Cremation:
Seven-year gap in resume. Skills atrophied. Network evaporated. References dated. Even if health improved, career couldn't recover. Lifetime earnings loss: Estimated $2.3 million.

The Insurance Illusion

Having insurance doesn't mean having healthcare:

The Deductible Doom:
$2,000 deductible. Sounds manageable. Hit by January 15th. Every year.

The Coinsurance Con:
After deductible, pay 20%. Sounds reasonable. 20% of 50,000surgeryis50,000surgeryis10,000. Not reasonable.

The Out-of-Pocket Joke:
$8,000 maximum out-of-pocket. Per year. For

in-network. Out-of-network unlimited. Specialists often out-of-network.

The Coverage Gaps:

- Dental separate (chronic illness affects teeth)
- Vision separate (medications affect eyes)
- Hearing separate (treatments cause hearing loss)
- Mental health limited
- Alternative treatments excluded

Insurance is financial shield made of Swiss cheese. Covers some things, leaves you exposed everywhere else.

The Medication Money Pit

The Branded Bankruptcy:
New medication, no generic: 1,200/monthInsurancecovers801,200/monthInsurancecovers80240/month
Need four medications: 960/monthAnnualmedicationcost:960/monthAnnualmedicationcost:11,520 AFTER insurance

The Generic Roulette:
Generic available but doesn't work same. Brand necessary but insurance refuses. Pay difference yourself or suffer.

The Formulary Shuffle:
Medication covered this year, not next. No warning. Discover at pharmacy. Scramble for alternatives or pay full price.

The Specialty Pharmacy Scam:
Must use specific pharmacy. Always more expensive. Often delayed. Sometimes "lost." No recourse.

The International Alternative:
Same medication in Canada:
100InUS:100InUS:1,000
Medical tourism for medication. Technically illegal. Frequently necessary.

The Credit Destruction

Medical debt destroys credit differently:

The Delayed Bombing:
Medical bills take months to arrive. By then, sent to collections. Credit score destroyed before you knew debt existed.

The Negotiation Nightmare:
Hospital says call insurance. Insurance says call hospital. Meanwhile, collections calling. Credit plummeting.

The Payment Plan Paradox:
Arrange payment plan with hospital. Hospital sells

debt anyway. Collections doesn't honor plan. Credit ruined despite trying.

My credit score:

- Before illness: 780
- After year one: 650
- After year three: 520
- After bankruptcy: 480

Can't rent apartment. Can't get car loan. Can't get credit card. Poverty becomes prison.

The Family Financial Fallout

The Spousal Sacrifice:
Mark's income became everything. His raise went to my medications. His bonus to my treatments. His dreams to my survival. Marriage became economic partnership where he contributed all, I consumed all.

The Parental Pauperization:
Parents liquidated retirement helping. Now they can't retire. My illness stole their future too.

The Sibling Strain:
Sister couldn't afford college because parents' savings went to my medical bills. My illness changed her life trajectory.

The Generational Theft:
No savings for potential children. No inheritance to leave. No generational wealth building. Illness creates poverty that echoes through generations.

The GoFundMe Generation

Medical crowdfunding is modern begging:

The Humiliation Arithmetic:
Writing your tragedy for public consumption. Posting photos at your worst. Begging friends for money. Watching fundraiser stall at 12% of goal.

My GoFundMe:

- Goal: $50,000
- Raised: $15,000
- Donors: 147
- Shares: 1,200
- Emotional cost: Immeasurable

Grateful for every dollar. Ashamed of needing it.

The Viral Lottery:
Successful campaigns need compelling story, attractive patient, social media savvy, network with money. Boring illnesses don't go viral. Ugly diseases don't get funded.

The Competition Cruelty:
35% of GoFundMe is medical. Competing with

children with cancer for stranger's dollars. Everyone deserving. Few funded.

The Financial Coping Strategies

The Bill Negotiation:

- Always ask for itemized bills
- Challenge every error (there are many)
- Request financial assistance (most hospitals required to offer)
- Negotiate payment plans
- Offer lump sum settlements
- Never ignore (makes worse)

Saved $30,000 through aggressive negotiation.

The Assistance Archaeology:

- Pharmaceutical company patient assistance
- Disease-specific foundations
- Local charities
- Religious organizations
- Government programs
- Hospital financial aid

Hours researching for every dollar saved. Part-time job being professionally poor.

The Strategic Default:
Sometimes bankruptcy is best option. Medical

bankruptcy doesn't make you failure — makes you survivor of failed system.

Considered bankruptcy year three. Lawyer said "You're perfect candidate." Decided to keep fighting. Maybe mistake.

The International Comparison

UK: NHS covers everything. Zero medical bankruptcy.
Canada: Universal healthcare. Medications separate but manageable.
Germany: Insurance covers all, including transportation.
Japan: Capped costs, extensive coverage.
USA: Leading cause of bankruptcy is medical debt.

American exceptionalism: Exceptionally cruel to sick people.

The Policy Solutions

Medicare for All:
Would eliminate most medical bankruptcy. Cost less than current system. Save 68,000 lives annually. Politically "impossible."

Public Option:
Government insurance competing with private.

Would lower costs, increase coverage. Still fought viciously.

Drug Price Controls:
Every other country negotiates drug prices. US forbidden by law. Pharma profits over patient lives.

Medical Debt Reform:
Eliminate credit reporting for medical debt. Cap interest rates. Require transparent pricing. Strengthen charity care requirements.

All possible. None happening. Because suffering is profitable.

The Financial Toxicity Support Network

Organizations Helping:

- RIP Medical Debt (buys and forgives debt)
- Patient Advocate Foundation (financial assistance)
- HealthWell Foundation (copay assistance)
- NeedyMeds (medication assistance)
- Dollar For (hospital bill forgiveness)

Online Communities:

- r/medical_debt (Reddit support)
- Facebook medical bill help groups
- Discord servers for financial navigation

- Collective knowledge powerful

The Employer Evolution (Barely) Beginning

Some employers recognizing financial toxicity:

Extended Sick Leave:
Beyond legal requirements. Protecting income during illness.

Supplemental Insurance:
Critical illness coverage. Hospital indemnity. Gap insurance.

Medical Travel Benefits:
Covering costs for specialists. Transportation assistance.

Flexible Spending Expansion:
Increased FSA limits. Carryover allowances.

But most employers still see sick employees as expendable.

The Personal Finance Rewrite

Chronic illness requires different financial planning:

Emergency Fund:
Not 3-6 months. Need 12-18 months. Out-of-pocket maximum plus living expenses.

Insurance Maximization:
Always hit FSA maximum. Choose PPO over HDHP if chronically ill. Understand every benefit.

Credit Protection:
Monitor constantly. Dispute aggressively. Document everything.

Assistance Preparation:
Know programs before crisis. Applications ready. Documentation organized.

Bankruptcy Readiness:
Understand options. Know lawyers. Protect what's protectable.

Planning for poverty while hoping for health.

The Financial Trauma Psychology

Financial toxicity creates specific trauma:

Worthlessness:
Society measures value in productivity. When you can't produce, you feel worthless.

Shame:
Asking for help humiliating. Each bill reminder reinforces failure.

Anxiety:
Every envelope potential crisis. Phone calls probably collections. Future seems impossible.

Relationship Strain:
Money fights destroy marriages. Financial dependence creates power imbalances.

Suicide Ideation:
Life insurance pays out. Death seems like financial solution. Dark mathematics.

Needed therapy for financial trauma specifically. Therapist said common but rarely addressed.

The Financial Manifesto

We demand:

1. **Healthcare as human right** — Not financial product
2. **Transparent pricing** — Know costs before treatment
3. **Capped out-of-pocket costs** — Based on income
4. **Eliminated medical debt** — Forgiveness not bankruptcy

5. **Universal prescription coverage** — Medications shouldn't bankrupt
6. **Paid medical leave** — Illness shouldn't mean income loss
7. **Disability benefits that sustain life** — Not poverty wages
8. **Credit protection from medical debt** — Healthcare shouldn't destroy credit
9. **Financial counseling with diagnosis** — Planning support included
10. **Recognition that financial toxicity kills** — Treat as medical emergency

The Truth About Financial Toxicity

It's not about poor planning or financial irresponsibility. It's about a system that profits from suffering, that charges premium prices for basic needs, that transforms healing into luxury item.

Financial toxicity is violence. It's forcing people to choose between medication and food. It's watching credit destroyed by cancer. It's selling homes to pay for surgery. It's dying because treatment costs too much.

My financial destruction from illness:

- Total cost: $706,000
- Recovery possibility: Never

- American dream: Dead
- Survival: Somehow

But also:

- Knowledge gained: Invaluable
- People helped: Hundreds
- System exposed: Necessarily
- Revolution joined: Absolutely

Your financial toxicity is not your fault. Your medical debt is not moral failing. Your bankruptcy is not character flaw. Your GoFundMe is not shameful.

The revolution happens when we stop accepting financial toxicity as inevitable. When we recognize that healthcare is human right, not consumer good. When we demand system that heals without bankrupting.

Keep fighting bills. Keep seeking assistance. Keep sharing costs. Keep surviving.

Your life is worth more than any bill. And someday, we'll have system that recognizes that.

That's how financial toxicity becomes revolution catalyst.

Chapter 13: Relationships in Crisis — When Illness Tests Every Bond

"Chronic illness is the relationship stress test nobody prepares for — revealing who'll stay when you have nothing to offer, who'll run when things get hard, and who you'll become when everything you were disappears."

The 75% Marriage Mortality Rate

Three out of four marriages don't survive chronic illness. Higher if the wife is sick (men leave more). The statistics are stark, but the reality is nuanced — relationships don't just end, they slowly suffocate under weight of exhaustion, resentment, and grief for the life you planned together.

Mark and I almost became statistics. Year three, sitting in couples therapy, him saying "I don't know how much more I can take," me saying "I wish you'd just leave so I could stop feeling guilty for destroying your life."

The therapist said: "You're both grieving the same loss — the relationship you thought you'd have. The question isn't whether you can return to that. It's whether you can build something new from what remains."

We're still building. Some days are construction, some demolition. Seven years later, we're neither the couple we were nor the one we planned to be. We're something harder, scarred, but somehow stronger — like bones that break and heal denser.

The Relationship Autopsy Stages

Stage 1: The Crisis Bond (Months 1-6)
Acute crisis creates intensity. Partners rally. "In sickness and health" feels noble. Adrenaline sustains impossible pace. Love feels proven through sacrifice.

Mark slept in hospital chairs, missed work for appointments, researched all night. We'd never been closer or more codependent.

Stage 2: The Reality Reckoning (Months 6-18)
Chronic means forever. Exhaustion accumulates. Resentment creeps in. Sex disappears. Conversations become medical updates. Date nights extinct. You're patient and caregiver, not partners.

We stopped touching. Not dramatically — gradually. Hugs became functional. Kisses perfunctory. Bodies became medical equipment, not sources of pleasure.

Stage 3: The Resentment Reservoir (Years 1-3)
Sick partner resents dependence. Healthy partner resents burden. Both resent illness. Neither can say it. Silence grows. Distance expands. Love remains but feels irrelevant.

I resented Mark's health, freedom, future. He resented my needs, limitations, consumption of his life. We loved each other while hating our life together.

Stage 4: The Breaking Point (Year 3-4)
Someone says "I can't do this anymore." Affairs happen (emotional if not physical). Separation discussed. Lawyers consulted. The relationship flatlines.

Mark apartment-hunted secretly. I planned how I'd manage alone. We were together but already apart.

Stage 5: The Decision (Variable)
Stay and rebuild or leave and grieve. Neither easy. Both valid. No right answer.

We chose rebuilding. Not from obligation but recognition: We still liked who the other was becoming through this hell. Not everyone does. That's okay.

The Sex Life Nobody Discusses

Chronic illness murders sex:

Physical Barriers:

- Pain makes touch unbearable
- Fatigue makes effort impossible
- Medications destroy libido
- Body changes destroy confidence
- Medical equipment mood killer

Psychological Barriers:

- Depression eliminates desire
- Body becomes medical object
- Partner becomes caregiver
- Vulnerability feels dangerous
- Rejection fear paralyzing

Relationship Barriers:

- Resentment blocks intimacy
- Roles feel inappropriate
- Time never right
- Energy never available
- Connection severed

Our sex life: Year one: Monthly. Year two: Quarterly. Year three: Annually. Year four: Never.

The therapist asked: "What if sex didn't mean intercourse? What if intimacy meant any connection that reminds you you're more than patient and caregiver?"

We rebuilt intimacy from scratch. Holding hands during TV. Foot massages. Shared showers. Slow dancing in kitchen. Eventually, adapted sex that worked for my body. Not previous sex life, but sex life nonetheless.

The Friend Exodus

Chronic illness is friendship filter:

The Disappearing Acts:
Can't commit to plans. Cancel repeatedly. Stop getting invited. Friendships atrophy from neglect.

Lost 80% of pre-illness friends. Not dramatically. Just faded.

The Discomfort Departures:
Your illness reminds them of mortality. Your limitations make them uncomfortable. Your reality is their fear.

Friends who couldn't handle my wheelchair. My fatigue. My reality. Their discomfort mattered more than our history.

The Comparison Casualties:
Their problems seem trivial compared to yours. Or your problems make theirs seem insignificant. Connection breaks.

"I shouldn't complain about my job when you can't work." Friendship needs equality. Illness creates imbalance.

The Energy Economics:
Maintaining friendships requires energy you don't have. Texting feels exhausting. Calling impossible. Visiting unthinkable.

Friendship requires investment I couldn't afford. Emotional bankruptcy.

The Identity Shifts:
You're no longer who they befriended. Shared activities impossible. Common ground eroded.

From athlete friend to sick friend. From career friend to disabled friend. From fun friend to depressing friend.

The Family Fractures

The Parent Problem:
Parents watching children suffer is specific hell. They help too much or not enough. Boundaries impossible.

My mother called hourly. Father withdrew completely. Both loved me. Neither knew how to help. Both methods hurt.

The Sibling Strain:
Healthy siblings get less attention. Sick sibling gets resources. Resentment inevitable.

My sister: "Everything is always about your illness." She wasn't wrong. How could it not be?

The Extended Extraction:
Cousins, aunts, uncles fade. Holidays skipped. Gatherings missed. Extended family becomes strangers.

Haven't seen cousins in five years. Too sick to travel. They stopped asking.

The In-Law Issues:
In-laws watch their child sacrifice. Blame you consciously or not. Relationship strained.

Mark's mother: "This isn't the life I wanted for him." Neither did I. Neither did he. Yet here we are.

The New Relationship Rules

We developed survival strategies:

Separate Identity Time:
Two hours daily where Mark wasn't caregiver, I

wasn't patient. Reading, hobbies, friends. Separately.

Relationship Hours:
Daily 30 minutes talking about anything except illness. Weather, books, dreams. Remembering we're humans.

Intimacy Scheduling:
Sounds unromantic. But scheduling ensures it happens. Wednesday is connection day. Whatever that means that week.

Respite Requirements:
Mark takes one weekend monthly completely off. I arrange other care. He needs life beyond illness.

Communication Protocols:
Weekly relationship check-in. What's working? What's not? What do you need? Honest, even when hurts.

Future Planning:
Dream together even if dreams changed. Adapted adventure still adventure. Modified dreams still dreams.

The Dating While Disabled Dilemma

For those single or newly single:

The Disclosure Dilemma:
When do you tell? First date (might scare away)? Third date (feels like lying)? When it's serious (feels like trap)?

The Inspiration Inspiration:
Being someone's inspiration porn. "You're so brave!" "I could never handle that!" Dating you makes them feel good about themselves.

The Caretaker Attraction:
Attracting people who want to save you. Codependent from start. Unhealthy dynamics baked in.

The Rejection Reality:
Many will run when learning you're sick. That's about them, not you. But still hurts.

The Adapted Activities:
Traditional dates might not work. Creative alternatives required. Not everyone flexible enough.

Friend Sarah's strategy: Discloses immediately in profile. "Chronically ill, still interesting." Filters out incompatible immediately.

The Workplace Relationship Wreckage

The Colleague Confusion:
Sick too much. Unreliable. Accommodation needs.

Colleagues resentful. Professional relationships strained.

The Boss Bind:
Need accommodation but fear discrimination. Disclosure risks career. Non-disclosure risks performance.

The Network Neglect:
Can't network after work. Miss conferences. Skip social events. Professional relationships atrophy.

Career relationships are transactional. When you can't deliver, they disappear. LinkedIn connection means nothing when you're disabled.

The Support Group Relationships

New relationships form in illness:

The Illness Friends:
Bond over shared suffering. Understand without explanation. Available at 3 AM. Literally lifesaving.

My friend Emma from support group knows me in ways Mark can't. We share darkness he's spared from.

The Mentor Relationships:
People further along journey. Providing roadmap. Hope embodied.

Patricia, diagnosed 10 years before me, showed survival possible. Her existence was medicine.

The Mentee Connections:
Helping newly diagnosed. Purpose through service. Meaning from suffering.

Helping others helped me. Their progress, my purpose. Their hope, my healing.

The Relationship Revolution Required

Healthcare Including Partners:
Partners at appointments. Caregiver support automatic. Couple therapy with diagnosis.

Workplace Recognition:
Partner illness as life event. Flexibility for caregiving. Support for employees with sick partners.

Social Support Systems:
Respite care accessible. Support groups for partners. Community care coordination.

Cultural Shift:
Recognizing illness affects relationships. Supporting adaptation. Celebrating different relationship models.

The Truth About Relationships and Illness

Chronic illness reveals relationship truth — stripping away pretense, comfort, assumption. What remains is either foundation strong enough to rebuild on or rubble to clear away.

Some relationships won't survive. That's not failure — it's recognition that some bonds break under pressure. Leaving doesn't make you bad person. Staying doesn't make you saint.

But relationships that survive transform. Become something deeper than healthy relationships can achieve. Intimacy forged in crisis. Love proven through persistence. Partnership tested and true.

Mark and I aren't same couple we were. We're battle-scarred veterans of war we didn't choose, fighting together against common enemy. Our love isn't romantic anymore — it's revolutionary. We're choosing each other daily despite everything trying to tear us apart.

The Relationship Manifesto

We declare that relationships in illness deserve:

1. **Recognition of unique challenges** — Not standard relationship advice

2. **Support for both partners** — Illness affects everyone
3. **Respite without guilt** — Breaks necessary, not selfish
4. **Intimacy adaptation support** — Sex therapy, accommodation education
5. **Financial assistance** — Relationship counseling covered
6. **Community support** — Not isolated struggle
7. **Workplace flexibility** — For both partners
8. **Different relationship models** — Not all traditional
9. **Celebration of persistence** — Staying together is achievement
10. **Permission to leave** — When relationship harms more than helps

Your relationships will change. Some will end. Some will evolve. Some will surprise you with their strength. All will teach you about human capacity for both cruelty and kindness.

The revolution happens when we stop expecting relationships to remain unchanged by illness. When we support adaptation instead of demanding normalcy. When we recognize that love sometimes means leaving and sometimes means staying when everything says go.

Fight for relationships worth saving. Release those that aren't. Build new ones that understand. Know that you're worthy of love, sick or well.

That's how relationships become revolution.

Part IV: Fighting Back

Chapter 14: Patient Advocacy — From Victim to Victor in Your Own Care

"Patient advocacy isn't about being difficult — it's about refusing to be disposable. It's recognizing that nobody will fight for your life as hard as you will, and that fighting for yourself is not selfish but survival."

The Awakening from Patient to Advocate

Day 732 of my illness, something shifted. Sitting in another dismissive appointment, being told again that my symptoms didn't make sense, something inside me stood up while my body remained seated.

"No," I said. Single word. Complete sentence. Revolutionary act.

The doctor looked startled. Patients don't say no. We comply, conform, collapse. But I was done being good patient if good meant dead patient.

"No, these symptoms are real. No, I won't accept 'we don't know' as final answer. No, I won't try another antidepressant when this isn't depression. No, I won't leave without plan."

That "no" began my transformation from patient to advocate. From victim of system to navigator of it. From passive recipient to active participant.

Patient advocacy isn't role you choose — it's necessity you accept when realize nobody else will save you.

The Advocacy Awakening Stages

Stage 1: The Polite Phase
"Sorry to bother you but..." Apologizing for existing. Minimizing symptoms to seem reasonable. Accepting whatever offered. Gratitude for crumbs.

Spent year one apologizing for taking up space in medical system. Thank you for seeing me. Sorry for complex symptoms. Whatever you think best.

Stage 2: The Research Rebellion

Google becomes medical school. PubMed your new homepage. You know more about condition than primary care. Still afraid to show it.

Year two printing studies, highlighting relevant parts, hesitantly suggesting, "I found this interesting article..."

Stage 3: The Assertive Arrival

Stop asking, start stating. "I need referral to specialist." Not "Could you maybe consider...?" Direct communication. Clear expectations.

Year three learned to say: "That's not acceptable. What are our other options?"

Stage 4: The Strategic Systematization

Advocacy becomes methodology. Documentation systems. Communication strategies. Network building. You're running campaign for your life.

Year four had binders, spreadsheets, scripts, strategies. Professional patient advocate for myself.

Stage 5: The Collective Consciousness

Your advocacy expands beyond yourself. Fighting for systemic change. Your battle becomes everyone's war.

Year five founded patient organization. Individual advocacy insufficient. System change required.

The Self-Advocacy Survival Toolkit

The Documentation Defense:

- Record everything (where legal)
- Photograph visible symptoms
- Log symptom patterns
- Save all correspondence
- Create paper trail
- Build evidence case

My documentation saved me from psychiatric commitment when doctor decided physical symptoms were psychosis. Evidence proved otherwise.

The Communication Commandments:

1. Be specific not general ("Pain at 8/10" not "hurts a lot")
2. Use medical terminology when known
3. State needs clearly ("I need pain management referral")
4. Set boundaries firmly ("I'm not comfortable with that")
5. Request clarification always ("Can you explain that?")
6. Confirm next steps explicitly ("So we're doing X, Y, Z")
7. Follow up relentlessly

The Question Queue:
Never attend appointment without questions written. Prioritized list. Won't remember when stressed.

My standard questions:

- What are all our options?
- What are risks/benefits of each?
- What happens if we do nothing?
- What would you do if family member?
- Can I have time to decide?
- Who else should I consult?

The Support Squad:
Never advocate alone when vulnerable. Bring witness. They remember when you can't, speak when you're silenced, fight when you're exhausted.

Mark became my advocate advocate. When I was too sick to fight, he fought for me.

The Second Opinion Strategy:
Second opinions aren't betrayal — they're due diligence. Different perspectives reveal different possibilities.

Got three opinions on surgery. First: Absolutely necessary. Second: Absolutely not. Third: Try conservative treatment first. Went with third. Avoided unnecessary surgery.

The System Navigation Masterclass

Understanding Power Dynamics:

- Doctors have medical knowledge
- You have body knowledge
- Insurance has financial power
- You have persistence power
- System has institutional authority
- You have moral authority

Leveraging Legislation:

- ADA requires reasonable accommodation
- HIPAA guarantees record access
- EMTALA prevents ER dumping
- Appeal rights for insurance denials
- State laws vary (know yours)

Finding Pressure Points:

- Patient satisfaction scores matter
- Online reviews have impact
- Complaints to medical boards noted
- Insurance commissioners have power
- Media attention changes everything

Building Your Network:

- Primary care quarterback
- Specialist team members

- Advocate allies
- Legal resources
- Political connections
- Media contacts

The Insurance Battle Tactics

The Appeal Arsenal:

- Never accept first denial
- Appeal immediately (deadlines matter)
- Include medical literature
- Get physician support letter
- Document financial hardship
- Threaten regulatory complaint
- Consider legal action

Won 23 of 34 appeals. Persistence pays.

The Prior Authorization Warfare:

- Request peer-to-peer review
- Demand reviewing physician credentials
- Record conversations
- Escalate to supervisors
- File complaints with insurance commission
- Share story publicly
- Name and shame

The Medical Record Revolution

Your Rights:

- Access all records
- Request amendments
- Add patient statements
- Correct errors
- Know who accessed
- Control sharing

Strategic Amendments:
Found "anxiety" throughout records. Added statement: "Patient's anxiety is appropriate response to medical trauma and diagnostic delay. Physical symptoms are not psychiatric."

Creating Alternate Record:
Keep your own medical record. Your perspective. Your truth. Your evidence.

The Appointment Advocacy

Pre-Appointment Power:

- Send agenda ahead
- Request appropriate time
- Research provider background
- Prepare documentation
- Plan your approach
- Practice difficult conversations

During-Appointment Authority:

- Lead with most important issue
- Redirect when dismissed
- Request specific actions
- Refuse inappropriate treatment
- Ask for everything in writing
- Stand your ground

Post-Appointment Action:

- Send summary email
- Correct any misunderstandings
- Follow up on promises
- Schedule next steps
- Review/rate publicly
- Share intelligence with others

The Collective Advocacy Evolution

Individual advocacy hits walls. Collective advocacy breaks them down.

Patient Organizations:
Joined three, founded one. Collective voice louder than individual whisper.

Political Engagement:
Testified at state legislature about insurance reform. Met with representatives. Shared story publicly. Policy changed slowly.

Media Mobilization:
Local news story about insurance denial. Went viral. Insurance reversed decision within 48 hours. Public pressure works.

Research Participation:
Joined patient advisory board for research study. Ensured patient perspective included. Changed study design.

Professional Partnerships:
Partnered with progressive physicians. Patient-physician alliance powerful. Changed clinic protocols.

The Advocacy Wins and Losses

Wins:

- Got correct diagnosis after seven years
- Won insurance coverage for "experimental" treatment
- Changed hospital policy on visitor restrictions
- Helped pass state legislation on prior authorization
- Connected hundreds to appropriate care
- Built network of advocating patients

Losses:

- Couldn't save friend from medical neglect
- Lost years to diagnostic delay
- Bankrupted despite advocacy
- Relationships destroyed by advocacy exhaustion
- Health worsened from advocacy stress
- Burned out repeatedly

Advocacy isn't free. Costs energy, relationships, health. But alternative is accepting unnecessary suffering.

The International Inspiration

UK Patient Champions:
Embedded in NHS. Formal role. Paid position. Patient perspective integrated.

Canadian Patient Partners:
Research requires patient involvement. Funding contingent on engagement. Patients as partners, not subjects.

Dutch Patient Experts:
Trained patient experts. Educate medical students. Consult on cases. Expertise recognized.

America: Patients as problems, not partners. We're changing that.

The Physician Perspective on Patient Advocates

Dr. Williams: "Initially, assertive patients frustrated me. Felt like challenge to authority. Then realized they're my best teachers. Now I love engaged patients. They make me better doctor."

Dr. Anderson: "Patient advocates save lives. They catch errors, provide context, ensure follow-through. Every patient should advocate. Every doctor should welcome it."

Not all doctors agree. Some see advocacy as threat. Those aren't doctors you want.

The Advocacy Training Ground

Communication Skills:

- Assertiveness training
- Negotiation tactics
- Public speaking
- Written communication
- Conflict resolution

Knowledge Building:

- Medical terminology
- Research literacy

- Legal rights
- Insurance systems
- Political process

Emotional Management:

- Boundary setting
- Stress management
- Trauma processing
- Anger channeling
- Resilience building

Strategic Thinking:

- System analysis
- Power mapping
- Campaign planning
- Network building
- Media engagement

The Advocacy Support System

Organizations:

- Patient Advocate Foundation
- National Patient Advocate Foundation
- Patient advocacy organizations by condition
- Legal aid societies
- Disability rights organizations

Online Communities:

- Twitter #PatientAdvocate
- Facebook advocacy groups
- Reddit support communities
- Discord real-time support
- LinkedIn professional advocates

Resources:

- Advocacy training programs
- Webinars and workshops
- Books and guides
- Templates and scripts
- Legal resources

The Advocacy Manifesto

We declare that patient advocacy is:

1. **Right not privilege** — Every patient deserves advocacy
2. **Expertise not interference** — We know our bodies
3. **Partnership not battle** — Working with providers who listen
4. **Necessity not choice** — Required for survival
5. **Skill that's learnable** — Anyone can advocate
6. **Community practice** — We advocate together
7. **System change catalyst** — Individual stories drive policy

8. **Exhausting but essential** — Worth the cost
9. **Revolutionary act** — Challenging power structures
10. **Love in action** — For ourselves and others

The Truth About Patient Advocacy

It shouldn't be necessary. In functioning healthcare system, patients wouldn't need to fight for appropriate care. But system is broken, and waiting for fix while suffering is death sentence.

Patient advocacy is:

- Exhausting when you're already exhausted
- Expensive in energy you don't have
- Necessary for survival
- Powerful when collective
- Revolutionary in impact

My advocacy journey:

- Started from desperation
- Evolved through education
- Strengthened through community
- Expanded beyond myself
- Continues despite exhaustion

Because every patient who advocates makes path easier for next patient. Every victory opens doors. Every story shared reduces isolation.

You can advocate. Start small. Say no. Ask questions. Request records. Bring support. Join groups. Share story. Fight back.

Your advocacy matters. Your voice has power. Your story drives change. Your fight helps everyone.

The revolution happens when patients stop accepting inadequate care. When we recognize our expertise. When we demand partnership not paternalism.

Advocate for yourself. Advocate for others. Advocate until advocacy isn't necessary.

That's how patient advocacy becomes healthcare revolution.

Chapter 15: Policy and Systemic Change — From Personal Battle to Political War

"Individual suffering is data point. Collective suffering is pattern. Pattern demands policy change. Policy change requires political power. Political power comes from stories that become statistics that become systems transformation."

The Pipeline from Patient to Policy

Seven years fighting for my own care taught me individual battles can't fix systemic failures. You can advocate perfectly, document meticulously, fight brilliantly, and still lose to system designed for your defeat.

The moment I understood this: Sitting in state legislature, testifying about prior authorization reform, watching insurance lobbyists outnumber patient advocates 10:1. They had money. We had stories. That day, money won.

But I learned something critical: Policy isn't made by people who understand problems — it's made by people with power. Patient advocates must become political advocates or accept perpetual suffering.

My pipeline from patient to policy maker:

- Year 1-3: Fighting for personal care
- Year 4: Joining patient organizations

- Year 5: Testifying at hearings
- Year 6: Meeting with legislators
- Year 7: Appointed to state health policy committee

From hospital bed to policy table. Because that's where decisions about our lives get made.

The American Healthcare Political Pathology

The Money Map:

- Insurance industry: $151 billion lobbying annually
- Pharmaceutical industry: $4.7 billion lobbying
- Hospital systems: $100 million lobbying
- Patient advocates: $0 (we're volunteers)

The Revolving Door:

- FDA commissioners become pharma executives
- Insurance executives become regulators
- Politicians' families on healthcare boards
- Conflict of interest everywhere

The Campaign Contribution Corruption:

- Average senator receives $500,000 from healthcare industry

- Key committee members receive millions
- Votes correlate with contributions
- Legal bribery determining policy

Wonder why healthcare reform fails? Follow the money.

The Levels of Change Required

Federal Level:

- Medicare for All (comprehensive solution)
- Public option (compromise position)
- Drug pricing reform (essential regardless)
- ACA protection/expansion (minimum requirement)
- NIH research prioritization (includes patients)

State Level:

- Insurance regulation (where real power lies)
- Medicaid expansion (lifesaving for millions)
- Surprise billing protection (state by state)
- Prescription drug boards (controlling costs)
- Patient rights legislation (varies wildly)

Local Level:

- Hospital charity care enforcement
- EMS policies

- Public health funding
- Community health centers
- Local ordinances (accessibility, etc.)

Institutional Level:

- Hospital policies
- Clinic procedures
- Insurance company practices
- Professional standards
- Medical education

Change needed everywhere simultaneously. Overwhelming? Yes. Necessary? Absolutely.

The Political Education of a Patient

Learning the Language:
Politics has different vocabulary than medicine. Had to learn:

- How bills become laws (Schoolhouse Rock lied)
- Committee structures (where bills die)
- Lobbying rules (barely any)
- Campaign finance (legalized corruption)
- Regulatory process (where details matter)

Understanding the Players:

- Elected officials (usually know nothing about healthcare)
- Staff members (actual power holders)
- Lobbyists (write the bills)
- Advocates (David vs. Goliath)
- Media (shapes narrative)

Recognizing the Games:

- Bills with nice names doing opposite
- Amendments that gut reform
- Procedural kills of good bills
- Industry-written "patient protection" acts
- Bipartisan agreement to do nothing

The Testimony That Changes Nothing and Everything

First time testifying at state legislature about prior authorization reform:

Prepared for weeks. Three minutes to condense seven years of suffering. Wore my best outfit to look "credible." Brought medical records as evidence.

Told story of nearly dying waiting for insurance approval. Committee members checked phones. Insurance lobbyist testified after me — suit worth more than my medical debt, spoke for 15 minutes about "fiscal responsibility."

Bill died in committee.

But: Reporter was there. Story ran. Other patients contacted me. We organized. Next year, we brought 50 patients. Year after, 200. Fourth year, bill passed.

Individual testimony rarely changes votes. Collective testimony changes narrative. Changed narrative changes policy. Eventually.

The Organizations Fighting

National:

- Patients for Affordable Drugs (drug pricing)
- Families USA (healthcare justice)
- National Patient Advocate Foundation (patient rights)
- Doctors for America (physician-patient alliance)
- Healthcare NOW (single-payer advocacy)

Disease-Specific:

- American Cancer Society (powerful lobby)
- Arthritis Foundation (active advocacy)
- National MS Society (research and access)
- Rare disease organizations (collective power)

Professional:

- Physicians for National Health Program (single-payer doctors)
- Nurses unions (powerful allies)
- Social workers associations (frontline fighters)

Joined five organizations. Power in numbers.

The Victories (Small but Significant)

State Level Wins:

- Prior authorization reform (modest but meaningful)
- Step therapy limitations (stopping forced medication fails)
- Insulin copay caps (lifesaving)
- Surprise billing protection (partial)
- Telehealth expansion (COVID silver lining)

Federal Progress:

- No Surprises Act (flawed but helpful)
- Drug pricing provisions in IRA (first step)
- ACA survival (multiple attempts to kill)
- Mental health parity enforcement (barely)
- Disabled access improvements (incremental)

Each victory took years, countless advocates, enormous energy. Incremental progress while people die waiting for transformation.

The Resistance and Backlash

Every patient protection faces industry opposition:

Their Tactics:

- "It will raise costs" (for their profits)
- "Reduce access" (to their control)
- "Hurt innovation" (their monopolies)
- "Government overreach" (into their corruption)
- "Socialism" (their nuclear option)

Their Weapons:

- Unlimited money
- Captured regulators
- Complicit politicians
- Media ownership
- Disinformation campaigns

Our Weapons:

- True stories
- Moral authority
- Growing numbers
- Social media
- Persistence despite everything

David vs. Goliath, if Goliath had billion-dollar budget and army of lobbyists.

The International Inspiration and Shame

What Works Elsewhere:

- UK: NHS provides universal coverage (flawed but functional)
- Canada: Single-payer works (with challenges)
- Germany: Multi-payer universal system (efficient)
- Japan: Cost controls and coverage (sustainable)
- Nordic countries: Healthcare as human right (revolutionary concept)

Why America Refuses:

- Profits over people
- Individualism mythology
- Regulatory capture
- Propaganda effectiveness
- Political cowardice

American exceptionalism: Exceptionally cruel to sick people, exceptionally profitable for corporations.

The COVID Catalyst

Pandemic revealed healthcare's failures:

Exposed:

- Employment-based insurance insanity
- Public health infrastructure collapse
- Inequality killing people
- Mental health crisis severity
- Essential workers' vulnerability

Temporary Solutions:

- Medicaid expansion
- Free vaccines
- Telehealth accessibility
- Eviction moratoriums
- Paid sick leave

Proved change possible when political will exists. Then political will evaporated. Back to normal dysfunction.

The Movement Building

Grassroots Growing:

- Patient story banks
- Coordinated testimony
- Social media campaigns
- Direct actions

- Electoral engagement

Coalition Construction:

- Patients + providers
- Labor + health advocates
- Faith communities + activists
- Business + workers
- Unusual alliances

Narrative Shifting:

- From individual responsibility to systemic failure
- From charity to rights
- From costs to investments
- From patients to people
- From profit to purpose

The Political Participation Prescription

For Beginners:

1. Register to vote (basic but essential)
2. Know your representatives (federal, state, local)
3. Join one organization (pick your issue)
4. Attend one meeting (see how it works)
5. Share your story (publicly, repeatedly)

For Intermediate:

1. Testify at hearings
2. Meet with legislators
3. Write op-eds
4. Organize others
5. Campaign for candidates

For Advanced:

1. Run for office
2. Lead organizations
3. Draft legislation
4. Build coalitions
5. Change systems

Started beginner. Now advanced. Every level matters.

The Personal Political Price

Political advocacy while chronically ill costs:

Energy:
Testifying exhausts. Organizing depletes. Fighting systems while fighting illness nearly impossible.

Money:
Travel to capitals. Time off work. Professional clothes. All unpaid.

Health:
Stress worsens symptoms. Disappointment hurts

physically. Victories temporary highs before crashes.

Relationships:
Political engagement strains relationships. Friends tire of advocacy. Family wants you to "just focus on getting better."

Hope:
Watching good bills die. Seeing corruption win. Knowing people die while politicians delay. Hope harder to maintain than health.

But alternative is accepting unnecessary suffering. That's unbearable.

The Policy Manifesto

We demand:

1. **Healthcare as human right** — Constitutional amendment
2. **Universal coverage** — Nobody uninsured
3. **Cost controls** — Healthcare shouldn't bankrupt
4. **Patient representation** — On every health board
5. **Transparent pricing** — Know costs upfront
6. **Mental health parity** — Actually enforced
7. **Prescription drug reform** — Affordable medications
8. **Research priorities** — Include patient input

9. **Provider protection** — From corporate medicine
10. **System transformation** — Not incremental tweaks

The Truth About Policy Change

It's slow. Frustrating. Corrupt. Seemingly impossible. But it's where power lives. Where decisions get made. Where suffering becomes statistics that sometimes spark change.

Individual advocacy saves individual lives. Policy advocacy saves everyone's lives.

My policy journey:

- Started angry at system
- Learned how system works
- Engaged despite exhaustion
- Small victories amid defeats
- Continue because must

Policy change requires:

- Stories becoming statistics
- Statistics becoming studies
- Studies becoming evidence
- Evidence becoming legislation
- Legislation becoming law
- Law becoming enforcement

- Enforcement becoming culture
- Culture becoming expectation

We're building movement. From hospital beds. From wheelchairs. From bankruptcy. From grief. From rage. From hope.

Every patient who votes advocates. Every story shared shapes narrative. Every testimony chips at fortress. Every victory opens doors.

The revolution happens when patients become political. When we stop accepting that healthcare is consumer good. When we demand that healing is human right.

Engage politically. Despite exhaustion. Despite cynicism. Despite everything.

Your story is political. Your suffering is political. Your survival is political. Your voice matters.

That's how patients become policy makers. That's how suffering becomes systemic change.

That's revolution.

Conclusion: The Revolution Will Be Humanized

"The revolution doesn't arrive with fanfare and flags. It begins in hospital rooms where patients say 'no more.' It builds in waiting rooms where strangers become allies. It spreads through stories that become movements. It succeeds when we stop accepting that suffering is inevitable and start demanding that healing is possible."

The View from Seven Years Later

As I write this conclusion, it's been 2,555 days since my body collapsed and my education in American healthcare began. Seven years of fighting for diagnosis, treatment, dignity, and change. Seven years that broke me and rebuilt me into someone I barely recognize — patient, advocate, revolutionary.

I'm writing from bed, where I spend 18 hours daily. My heart rate monitor beeps steadily at 95 (lying down). Morning medications — all 11 of them — wait in their weekly organizer. The shower chair is positioned for when I have energy to bathe. Mark is downstairs working, earning the income that keeps us housed and insured.

By any traditional measure, I'm defeated. Career destroyed. Savings depleted. Body broken. Dreams deferred.

But traditional measures miss the revolution happening in this room, in thousands of rooms, where patients are transforming from victims to victors, from statistics to storytellers, from problems to solutions.

We're not waiting for healthcare to be fixed. We're fixing it ourselves, one story, one connection, one small victory at a time.

What Has Changed

In Medicine:

- Patient experience finally being measured
- Shared decision-making gaining ground
- Telehealth expanding access
- Chronic illness recognition growing
- Mental health integration beginning
- Patient advisors in some hospitals
- Medical education including patient voices

Not enough. Not fast enough. But movement.

In Technology:

- Apps connecting patients
- AI assisting diagnosis
- Wearables tracking symptoms
- Online communities thriving
- Information democratizing
- Telemedicine normalizing
- Digital health exploding

Technology isn't salvation but it's enabling revolution.

In Culture:

- Chronic illness visibility increasing
- Disability representation improving
- Patient stories being heard
- Medical gaslighting being named
- Health equity discussions mainstream
- Pandemic revealing systemic failures
- Younger generations demanding better

Culture shifts slowly, then suddenly. We're approaching suddenly.

In Policy:

- Incremental insurance reforms
- Drug pricing attention
- Surprise billing protection
- Mental health parity enforcement
- Telehealth reimbursement
- Patient advocacy recognition
- State-level experiments

Baby steps when we need giant leaps, but steps nonetheless.

What Hasn't Changed (Yet)

- Healthcare still tied to employment
- Insurance companies still denying care
- Medications still bankrupting families
- Doctors still interrupting after 11 seconds
- ERs still traumatizing
- Diagnoses still taking years
- Mental health still separated from physical
- Caregivers still invisible
- Alternative medicine still desperate last resort
- Medical debt still destroying lives
- Relationships still fracturing
- Advocacy still exhausting
- Politics still corrupted
- Profit still prioritized over people

The foundation remains rotten even as we patch cracks.

The Lessons Learned

Personal Lessons:

1. Your body knows things medicine hasn't discovered

2. Advocacy is survival skill, not personality trait
3. Community heals what medicine can't
4. Boundaries are medical necessities
5. Hope requires constant cultivation
6. Suffering can become purpose
7. Survival is resistance
8. Rest is revolutionary
9. Your story matters
10. You're stronger than you know

Systemic Lessons:

1. Individual solutions can't fix systemic problems
2. Patient expertise is real expertise
3. Profit-driven healthcare is oxymoron
4. Insurance companies practice medicine without licenses
5. Political will creates immediate change
6. Collective action works
7. Stories change policy
8. Money corrupts medicine
9. Other countries prove better is possible
10. Revolution is necessary

The People Who Made This Possible

This book exists because:

- Mark never left when staying seemed impossible
- Dr. Chen listened when others dismissed
- Sarah attended appointments as witness
- Emma from support group texted at 3 AM
- Patricia showed survival was possible
- Mom liquidated retirement to help
- Hundreds of patients shared their stories
- Progressive doctors fight alongside us
- Advocates dedicate lives to change
- You picked up this book

Revolution requires community. Nobody survives alone.

The Call to Revolution

To Patients:
Your suffering is not your fault. Your expertise is valid. Your story needs telling. Your advocacy matters. Join us.

To Families:
Your exhaustion is real. Your sacrifice seen. Your needs matter. Your limits valid. You deserve support.

To Providers:
Your compassion is medicine. Your listening heals. Your partnership transforms. Your advocacy amplifies. Join the revolution from inside.

To Policy Makers:
Your decisions determine lives. Your courage creates change. Your resistance kills. Choose wisely. History is watching.

To Everyone:
You will be patient eventually. This is your fight too. Start now while you have energy. Build the system you'll need.

The Revolution Roadmap

Individual Level:

1. Share your story
2. Connect with others
3. Advocate for yourself
4. Support fellow patients
5. Educate yourself
6. Set boundaries
7. Find purpose in pain
8. Build sustainable life
9. Maintain hope
10. Keep fighting

Community Level:

1. Join support groups
2. Create mutual aid networks
3. Share resources
4. Amplify voices
5. Organize locally

6. Support caregivers
7. Challenge stigma
8. Build alternative systems
9. Celebrate victories
10. Sustain each other

System Level:

1. Demand universal healthcare
2. Regulate insurance industry
3. Control drug prices
4. Integrate mental health
5. Support caregivers
6. Fund research properly
7. Include patient voices
8. Measure what matters
9. Prioritize prevention
10. Value health over wealth

The Future We're Building

Imagine healthcare where:

- Nobody goes bankrupt from illness
- Insurance covers everything necessary
- Medications are affordable
- Appointments last as long as needed
- Doctors listen fully
- Mental health is included
- Caregivers are supported
- Alternative medicine is integrated
- Patient expertise is valued

- Dignity is guaranteed
- Healing is human right

This isn't utopian fantasy. Other countries approach this. We can too. We must.

The Personal Postscript

Would I choose this journey? Never. Am I grateful for who it's made me? Surprisingly, yes.

I've learned that:

- Horizontal is position, not defeat
- Productivity doesn't determine worth
- Weakness reveals strength
- Vulnerability creates connection
- Suffering can generate purpose
- Small victories matter immensely
- Community is medicine
- Hope is discipline
- Survival is success
- Revolution happens in bed

My body may be broken, but my spirit is steel forged in medical fire. My career may be over, but my purpose is clear. My old life is dead, but my new life has meaning.

This isn't inspiration porn. This is recognition that we can transform poison into medicine, suffering into service, patients into revolutionaries.

The Final Prescription

Take daily:

- One dose of righteous anger
- Multiple tablets of mutual support
- Continuous infusion of hope
- Regular injections of advocacy
- Unlimited refills of community
- As-needed doses of rest
- Scheduled boundaries
- Chronic courage
- Persistent resistance
- Revolutionary love

Side effects include: System change, dignity, justice, healing, transformation.

No prior authorization required.

The Last Word (Which Is Really the First)

This book began with me on yoga mat, unable to keep up, told "maybe this isn't for you." That instructor was wrong. This is for me. For all of us. Healthcare, dignity, support, change — it's all for us.

We're not asking for special treatment. We're demanding human treatment. We're not seeking charity. We're requiring justice. We're not begging for help. We're building new systems.

The revolution has already begun. In support groups sharing resources. In exam rooms where patients say no. In legislatures where we testify. In communities where we care for each other. In beds where we refuse to surrender.

We are millions strong. We are patients, caregivers, providers, humans. We are exhausted but persistent. We are broken but building. We are suffering but surviving.

And we will not stop until healthcare is human right, until dignity is guaranteed, until healing is possible for all.

The revolution will not be televised. It will be humanized. It will happen in hospitals and homes, in congress and communities, in individual hearts and collective action.

It has already begun.

Join us.

Your life depends on it.

All our lives depend on it.

Welcome to the revolution.

End of "What Do Patients Want: A Revolutionary Guide to Healthcare Transformation Through Partnership"

For resources, references, and continued revolution, visit: chronically.life

Share your story: hi@chronically.life

Join the movement: Chronically

Remember: You are not alone. You are not crazy. You are not beyond hope.

You are revolutionary.

www.ingramcontent.com/pod-product-compliance
Lightning Source LLC
Chambersburg PA
CBHW052343220526
45465CB00003BA/939